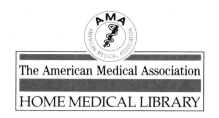

The American Medical Association

HOME MEDICAL LIBRARY

PREGNANCY AND CHILDBIRTH

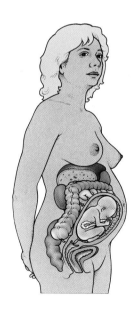

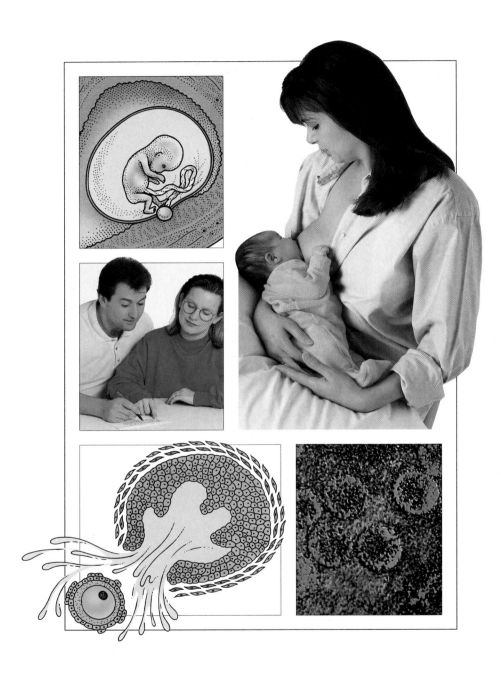

THE AMERICAN
MEDICAL ASSOCIATION

PREGNANCY
AND
CHILDBIRTH

Medical Editor
CHARLES B. CLAYMAN, MD

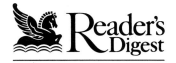

THE READER'S DIGEST ASSOCIATION, INC.
Pleasantville, New York/Montreal

The AMA Home Medical Library was created and produced
by Dorling Kindersley, Ltd., in association with the
American Medical Association.

The information in this book reflects current medical knowledge. The
recommendations and information are appropriate in most cases;
however, they are not a substitute for medical diagnosis. For specific
information concerning your personal medical condition, the AMA
suggests that you consult a physician.

The names of organizations, products, or alternative therapies appearing
in this book are given for informational purposes only. Their inclusion
does not imply AMA endorsement, nor does the omission of any
organization, product, or alternative therapy indicate AMA disapproval.

The AMA Home Medical Library is distinct from and unrelated to the
series of health books published by Random House, Inc., in conjunction
with the American Medical Association under the names "The AMA Home
Reference Library" and "The AMA Home Health Library."

Library of Congress Cataloging in Publication Data

Pregnancy and childbirth / medical editor, Charles B. Clayman.
     p.   cm. — (The American Medical Association home medical
library)
  At head of title: The American Medical Association.
  Includes index.
  ISBN 0-89577-465-8
  1. Pregnancy.   2. Childbirth.   I. Clayman, Charles B.
II. American Medical Association.   III. Series.
RG525.P6786 1993
618.2—dc20   92-21988

FOREWORD

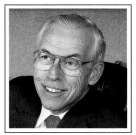

Having a baby is – and has always been – one of life's most precious miracles, but this experience has changed tremendously over the years. One of the most notable changes is that women today are better informed about what to expect during pregnancy and better prepared to cope with the demands of labor and delivery. Also, because of advances in technology and an ever-increasing understanding of the processes of pregnancy and childbirth, a woman's chances of having a trouble-free pregnancy and a healthy baby are better than ever before.

The time to start planning for your baby is before you conceive. Eating a well-balanced diet, getting plenty of exercise, and enjoying a healthy life-style will help ensure a healthy pregnancy and give your baby the best possible start in life. Once you become pregnant, continuing these habits and getting early and regular prenatal care are essential.

In this volume, we help you prepare for pregnancy, discuss how your body changes and some temporary discomforts you may experience, describe the stages of development of the fetus, and explain the processes of labor and delivery. Although most pregnancies progress normally and end with the birth of a healthy baby, complications do sometimes occur. We discuss some of the problems that can develop and the types of medical intervention that may be needed during labor and delivery. In the final section, we discuss some of the causes of infertility and explain how the advances made in the treatment of this problem offer hope to many couples.

Whether you are a parent-to-be or are expecting the arrival of a grandchild or niece or nephew, we at the American Medical Association hope this volume of the Home Medical Library answers all your questions about pregnancy and childbirth.

James S Todd MD

JAMES S. TODD, MD
Executive Vice President
American Medical Association

CONTENTS

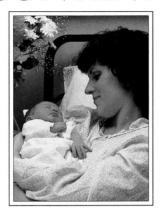

CHAPTER ONE

THE START OF A NEW LIFE

INTRODUCTION

THE REPRODUCTIVE
PROCESS

PLANNING FOR
PREGNANCY

YOUR CHANCES of having a healthy baby are better than ever before – thanks to advances in medical technology, emphasis on early and comprehensive prenatal care, and awareness of the importance of a healthy life-style. Research continues to investigate ways to reduce the rate of infant deaths in the US, which is one of the highest among developed countries. Perinatal mortality (the rate of stillbirths plus the rate of infant deaths occurring during the first week after birth) declined by 50 percent between 1950 and 1980 and continues to decrease. In addition, the rate of maternal deaths went down by 32 percent between 1979 and 1986. Medical researchers have identified many of the causes of abnormal fetal development and the disorders that can be harmful to a fetus. As a result, both doctors and parents-to-be have become much better prepared to help prevent these problems. Pregnancy starts when a man's sperm fertilizes a woman's egg. Although this is the beginning of the miracle of bringing a child into the world, you should begin preparing for pregnancy long before this moment. Having a baby brings many changes to a couple's life. You and your partner should discuss the adjustments you will need to make financially and socially. You both must

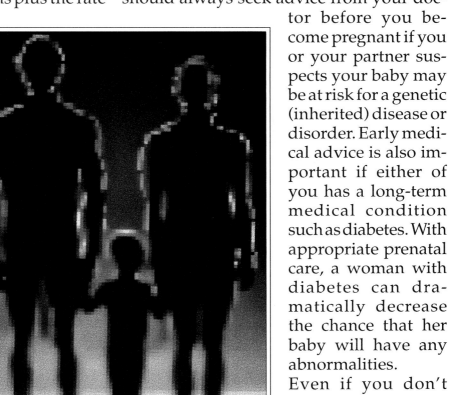

take an active role in ensuring the birth of a healthy baby by making sensible choices about your health and life-style. To give your baby a healthy start in life, talk to your doctor before you become pregnant about the positive steps you can take immediately (such as eating a well-balanced diet and staying physically fit, as well as stopping smoking and abstaining from alcohol). You should always seek advice from your doctor before you become pregnant if you or your partner suspects your baby may be at risk for a genetic (inherited) disease or disorder. Early medical advice is also important if either of you has a long-term medical condition such as diabetes. With appropriate prenatal care, a woman with diabetes can dramatically decrease the chance that her baby will have any abnormalities.

Even if you don't anticipate having any problems, you should make an appointment to see your doctor as soon as you think you might be pregnant. The first 3 months of pregnancy are very important because all of the baby's major organs develop during this time. Women who get medical care early in their pregnancies – and who return for regularly scheduled visits – are less likely to have medical problems during their pregnancies and are more likely to have healthy babies.

THE REPRODUCTIVE PROCESS

Humans reproduce by a process in which two cells (a woman's ovum, or egg, and a man's sperm) join. The union of these two cells, called fertilization, is the starting point for the development and birth of a new human being. The new, unique individual inherits half of his or her genetic characteristics from the woman's egg and half from the man's sperm.

The anatomy and functions of the reproductive organs in humans enable a sperm to fertilize an egg inside a woman's body. The fertilized egg is nourished and develops from a tiny embryo into a fetus. The fetus grows and matures in the uterus until it is able to survive outside the woman's body.

Human reproduction involves a remarkable series of processes in both the man and the woman. The functions of the reproductive organs of men and women and the process of fertilization are described in the following pages.

Diverse ways to reproduce
Not all species give birth to live offspring as mammals do. For example, after mating, the female bird lays eggs that have been fertilized by the male; young chicks develop inside a protective eggshell – outside the female's body.

FEMALE REPRODUCTIVE ORGANS

The organs that make up the female reproductive system (called the genital organs) have the capacity to produce and nourish eggs, enabling a new life to be created.

Ovary
Each ovary is a flat, almond-shaped gland, about 1 1/4 inches in length. The ovaries produce the hormones estrogen and progesterone and contain the tissue sacs called follicles in which eggs develop.

Location of the female reproductive organs
The drawing below shows the female reproductive organs in relation to other internal structures of a woman's abdomen.

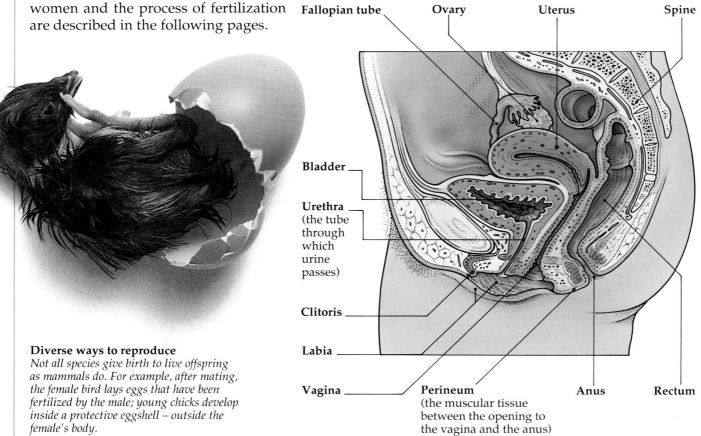

Fallopian tube   Ovary   Uterus   Spine

Bladder

Urethra (the tube through which urine passes)

Clitoris

Labia

Vagina   Perineum (the muscular tissue between the opening to the vagina and the anus)   Anus   Rectum

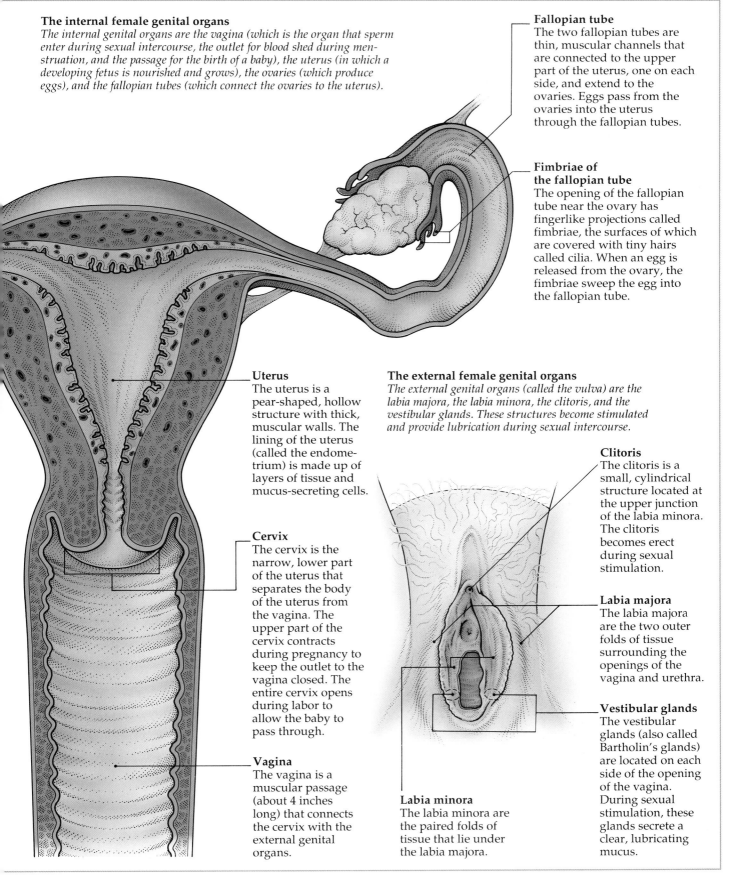

The internal female genital organs
The internal genital organs are the vagina (which is the organ that sperm enter during sexual intercourse, the outlet for blood shed during menstruation, and the passage for the birth of a baby), the uterus (in which a developing fetus is nourished and grows), the ovaries (which produce eggs), and the fallopian tubes (which connect the ovaries to the uterus).

Fallopian tube
The two fallopian tubes are thin, muscular channels that are connected to the upper part of the uterus, one on each side, and extend to the ovaries. Eggs pass from the ovaries into the uterus through the fallopian tubes.

Fimbriae of the fallopian tube
The opening of the fallopian tube near the ovary has fingerlike projections called fimbriae, the surfaces of which are covered with tiny hairs called cilia. When an egg is released from the ovary, the fimbriae sweep the egg into the fallopian tube.

Uterus
The uterus is a pear-shaped, hollow structure with thick, muscular walls. The lining of the uterus (called the endometrium) is made up of layers of tissue and mucus-secreting cells.

The external female genital organs
The external genital organs (called the vulva) are the labia majora, the labia minora, the clitoris, and the vestibular glands. These structures become stimulated and provide lubrication during sexual intercourse.

Clitoris
The clitoris is a small, cylindrical structure located at the upper junction of the labia minora. The clitoris becomes erect during sexual stimulation.

Cervix
The cervix is the narrow, lower part of the uterus that separates the body of the uterus from the vagina. The upper part of the cervix contracts during pregnancy to keep the outlet to the vagina closed. The entire cervix opens during labor to allow the baby to pass through.

Labia majora
The labia majora are the two outer folds of tissue surrounding the openings of the vagina and urethra.

Vestibular glands
The vestibular glands (also called Bartholin's glands) are located on each side of the opening of the vagina. During sexual stimulation, these glands secrete a clear, lubricating mucus.

Vagina
The vagina is a muscular passage (about 4 inches long) that connects the cervix with the external genital organs.

Labia minora
The labia minora are the paired folds of tissue that lie under the labia majora.

11

HOW EGGS ARE PRODUCED

When a female is born, her ovaries contain between 700,000 and 2 million ova (eggs) – a lifetime's supply. Each of these eggs – called a primary oocyte – is surrounded by a layer of cells called the granulosa cells. The entire structure is called a primary follicle. Most of the primary follicles gradually degenerate before a female reaches puberty. At the start of puberty, between 200,000 and 400,000 primary follicles remain.

At puberty, hormonal changes start to occur about every 28 days that stimulate up to 25 of the primary follicles to begin to mature into secondary follicles; only one primary follicle (occasionally two) reaches full maturation each month and releases a secondary oocyte from the ovary. This process is called ovulation.

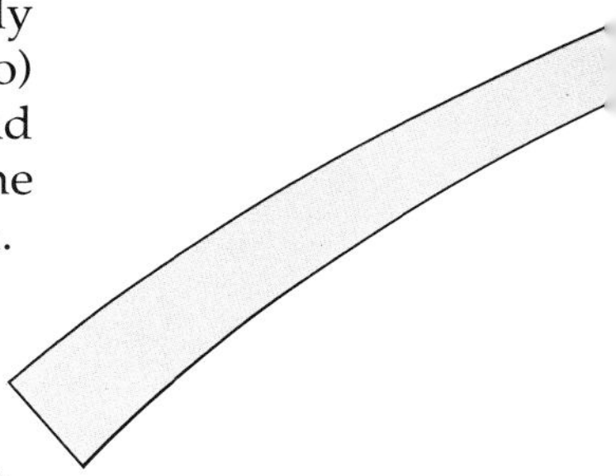

MATURATION AND RELEASE OF THE EGG

When a female reaches puberty, the pituitary gland, located at the base of the brain, begins to periodically secrete increased levels of follicle-stimulating hormone (FSH) and luteinizing hormone (LH). These hormones, which reach the ovaries through the bloodstream, coordinate the maturation of an egg and its release from the ovary (called ovulation).

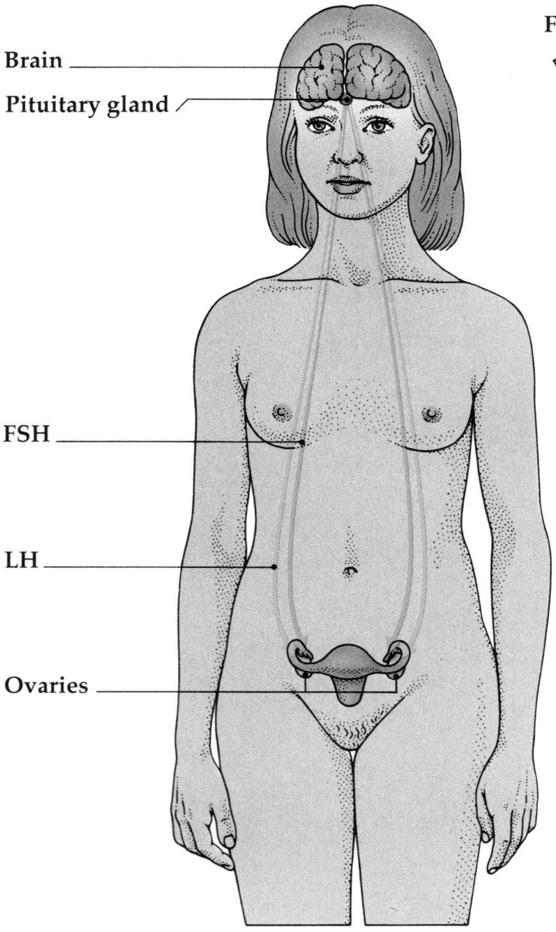

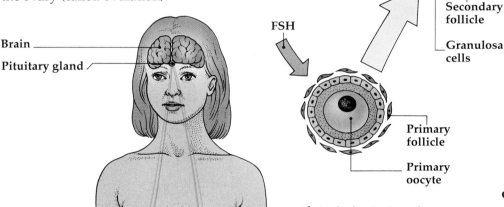

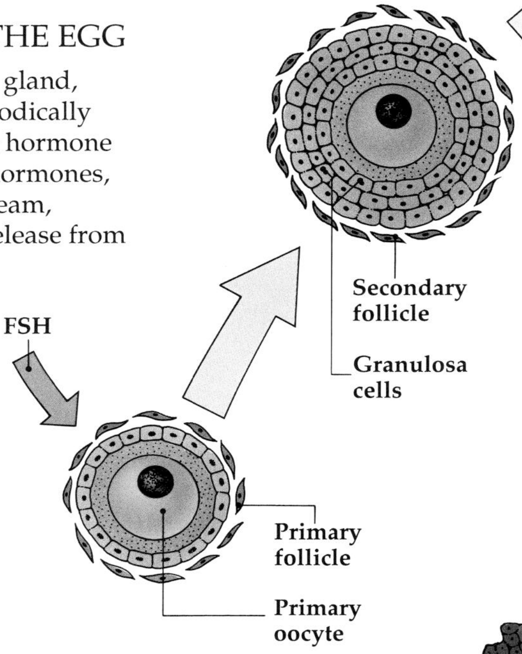

FSH

Secondary follicle

Granulosa cells

2 The maturing primary follicle enlarges as the cells surrounding the primary oocyte (called the granulosa cells) multiply and form several layers. This multilayered structure is now called a secondary follicle.

Primary follicle

Primary oocyte

Brain

Pituitary gland

FSH

LH

Ovaries

1 At the beginning of the menstrual cycle (see page 13), follicle-stimulating hormone (FSH) produced by the pituitary gland stimulates the growth of some of the primary follicles (which contain primary oocytes) in the ovaries. Usually only one primary follicle will reach the final stage of maturation.

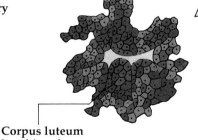

Corpus luteum breaking down

7 If fertilization occurs (see page 16), the corpus luteum continues to secrete hormones throughout the pregnancy. If fertilization does not occur, the corpus luteum starts to break down 10 to 12 days after the egg is released.

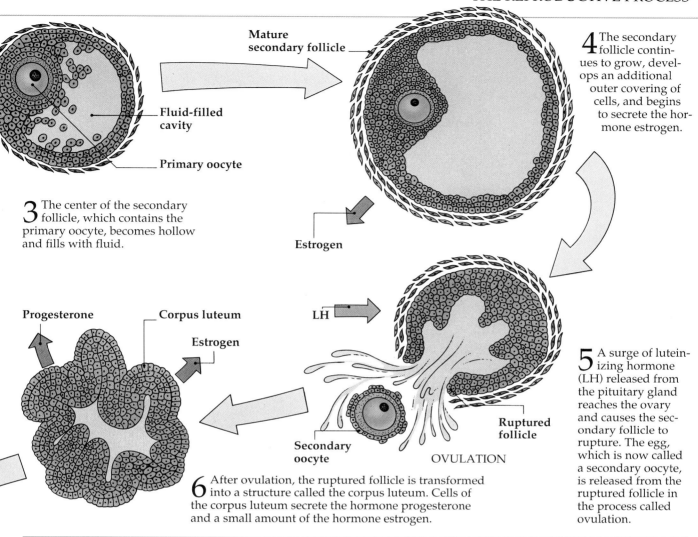

Mature secondary follicle

Fluid-filled cavity

Primary oocyte

3 The center of the secondary follicle, which contains the primary oocyte, becomes hollow and fills with fluid.

Estrogen

4 The secondary follicle continues to grow, develops an additional outer covering of cells, and begins to secrete the hormone estrogen.

Progesterone

Corpus luteum

Estrogen

LH

Ruptured follicle

Secondary oocyte

OVULATION

5 A surge of luteinizing hormone (LH) released from the pituitary gland reaches the ovary and causes the secondary follicle to rupture. The egg, which is now called a secondary oocyte, is released from the ruptured follicle in the process called ovulation.

6 After ovulation, the ruptured follicle is transformed into a structure called the corpus luteum. Cells of the corpus luteum secrete the hormone progesterone and a small amount of the hormone estrogen.

MENSTRUAL CYCLE

Changes in the uterus
Menstruation is the shedding of the lining of the uterus (called the endometrium) about every 28 days. The menstrual cycle functions so that when a woman ovulates, her uterus is prepared to nourish an embryo if one of her eggs is fertilized. If fertilization does take place, she will not have menstrual cycles during pregnancy.

1 Menstruation, the period of vaginal bleeding that occurs when the endometrium breaks down and is shed, lasts from day 1 to day 4 or 5 of the cycle.

2 Following menstruation, the hormone estrogen is released from the follicles in the ovaries and causes the endometrium to begin to thicken before ovulation occurs.

3 Ovulation usually occurs around day 15 of the cycle. Increased production of progesterone and estrogen stimulates further thickening of the endometrium.

4 If fertilization does not occur, progesterone and estrogen levels decrease. The endometrium breaks down after day 24 or 25 and is shed.

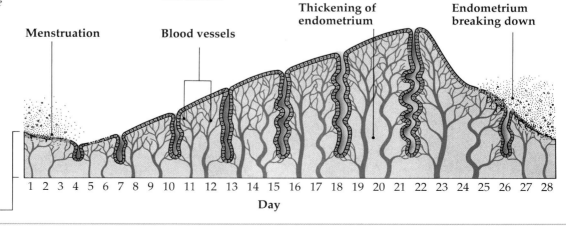

Menstruation

Blood vessels

Thickening of endometrium

Endometrium breaking down

Endometrium

1 2 3 4 5 6 7 8 9 10 11 12 13 14 15 16 17 18 19 20 21 22 23 24 25 26 27 28

Day

MALE REPRODUCTIVE ORGANS

The male reproductive organs include the testicles (in which sperm are produced), the vas deferens (which carries sperm from each testicle to the urethra – the tube through which urine and semen pass from the body), the seminal vesicles and the prostate and bulbo-urethral glands (which produce most of the fluids, called seminal fluid, that mix with sperm to form semen), and the penis (from which sperm are ejaculated during sexual intercourse).

Vas deferens
The vas deferens is the tube that carries sperm released from each testicle. Each vas deferens passes up and over the bladder and joins a seminal vesicle to form an ejaculatory duct at the upper part of the urethra.

Prostate gland
The prostate gland surrounds the upper part of the urethra, just below the bladder. This gland produces about 30 percent of the seminal fluid, which enters the urethra through many tiny ducts.

Bulbourethral glands
The bulbourethral glands are located on either side of the base of the penis. These glands produce about 5 percent of the seminal fluid.

Urethra
The urethra extends from the bladder to the end of the penis. The upper part of the urethra connects to each vas deferens. The urethra is the tube through which urine and semen are excreted from the body.

Testicles
The testicles are oval-shaped organs that produce sperm, the hormone testosterone, and about 5 percent of the seminal fluid.

Scrotum
The scrotum, a thin layer of skin over a layer of muscle, forms the pouch that contains the testicles.

Bladder

Seminal vesicle
Near the top of each vas deferens is a pouchlike gland called a seminal vesicle. These glands produce about 60 percent of the seminal fluid.

Ejaculatory duct
Each ejaculatory duct joins a seminal vesicle to a vas deferens and enters the upper part of the urethra.

Penis
The penis contains three columns of erectile tissue (spongy tissue full of tiny blood vessels – see SEXUAL AROUSAL IN A MAN below). The urethra runs through the center of one of the columns of tissue to the end of the penis.

Epididymis
The epididymis is a long, cordlike structure (lying along the back of each testicle) that opens into a vas deferens. Sperm mature and are stored in the epididymis.

Sexual arousal in a man
Sexual arousal in a man causes nerve impulses to stimulate the arteries that supply blood to the tissues of the penis. These arteries dilate (widen) and the tissue in the shaft of the penis, called erectile tissue, fills with blood. This buildup of blood causes the penis to increase in size and become erect, enabling it to enter the vagina.

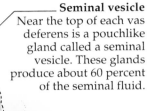

HOW SPERM ARE PRODUCED

Sperm production starts at puberty. A healthy man produces nearly 100 million sperm every day (about 1,000 sperm per second).

1 Sperm are produced and undergo the early stages of their development in the seminiferous tubules of the testicles. Clusters of cells in the tissue surrounding these tubules secrete the hormone testosterone, which is necessary for production and development of sperm.

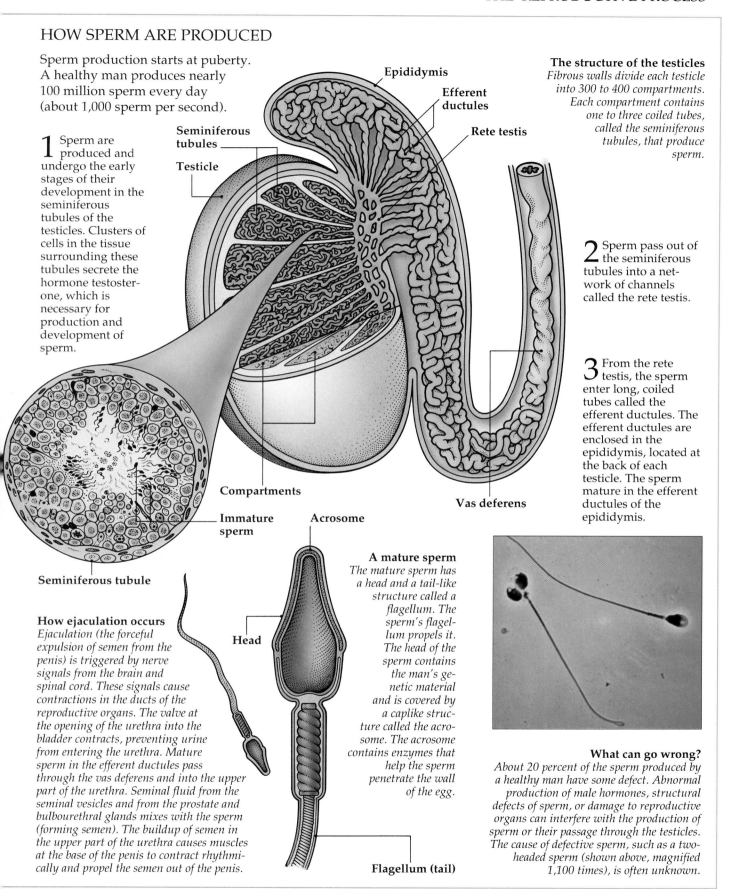

Epididymis

Efferent ductules

Rete testis

Seminiferous tubules

Testicle

Compartments

Immature sperm

Acrosome

Head

Seminiferous tubule

Vas deferens

Flagellum (tail)

The structure of the testicles
Fibrous walls divide each testicle into 300 to 400 compartments. Each compartment contains one to three coiled tubes, called the seminiferous tubules, that produce sperm.

2 Sperm pass out of the seminiferous tubules into a network of channels called the rete testis.

3 From the rete testis, the sperm enter long, coiled tubes called the efferent ductules. The efferent ductules are enclosed in the epididymis, located at the back of each testicle. The sperm mature in the efferent ductules of the epididymis.

How ejaculation occurs
Ejaculation (the forceful expulsion of semen from the penis) is triggered by nerve signals from the brain and spinal cord. These signals cause contractions in the ducts of the reproductive organs. The valve at the opening of the urethra into the bladder contracts, preventing urine from entering the urethra. Mature sperm in the efferent ductules pass through the vas deferens and into the upper part of the urethra. Seminal fluid from the seminal vesicles and from the prostate and bulbourethral glands mixes with the sperm (forming semen). The buildup of semen in the upper part of the urethra causes muscles at the base of the penis to contract rhythmically and propel the semen out of the penis.

A mature sperm
The mature sperm has a head and a tail-like structure called a flagellum. The sperm's flagellum propels it. The head of the sperm contains the man's genetic material and is covered by a caplike structure called the acrosome. The acrosome contains enzymes that help the sperm penetrate the wall of the egg.

What can go wrong?
About 20 percent of the sperm produced by a healthy man have some defect. Abnormal production of male hormones, structural defects of sperm, or damage to reproductive organs can interfere with the production of sperm or their passage through the testicles. The cause of defective sperm, such as a two-headed sperm (shown above, magnified 1,100 times), is often unknown.

FERTILIZATION OF AN EGG

Pregnancy begins with the union of an egg and a sperm (the process called fertilization), followed by the implantation of the fertilized egg in the wall of the uterus (known as conception).

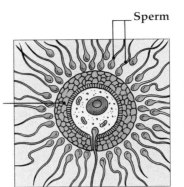

Sperm

Outer covering of egg

2 Only about 200 sperm survive the rest of the journey and reach the upper part of the fallopian tube, where fertilization occurs.

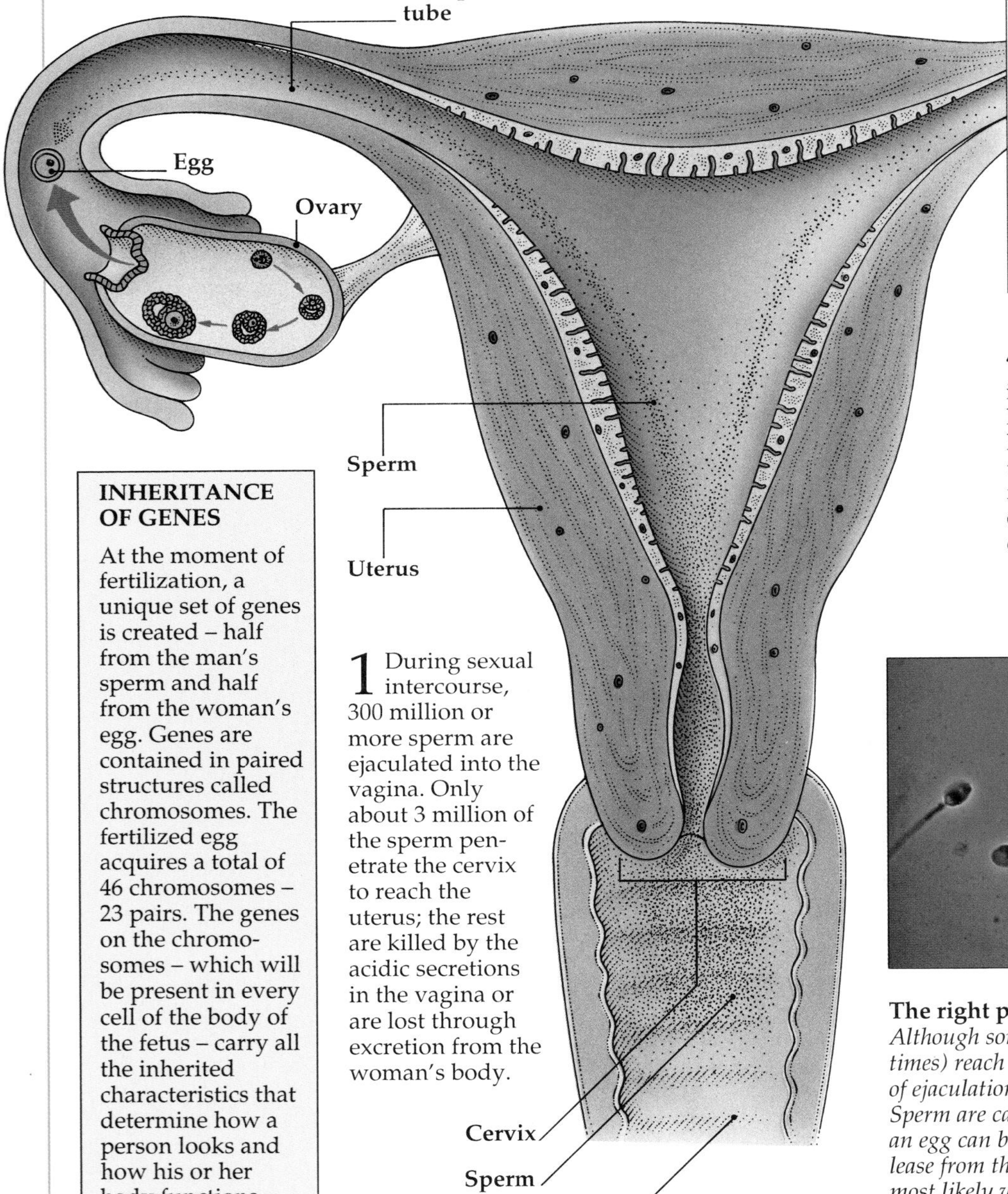

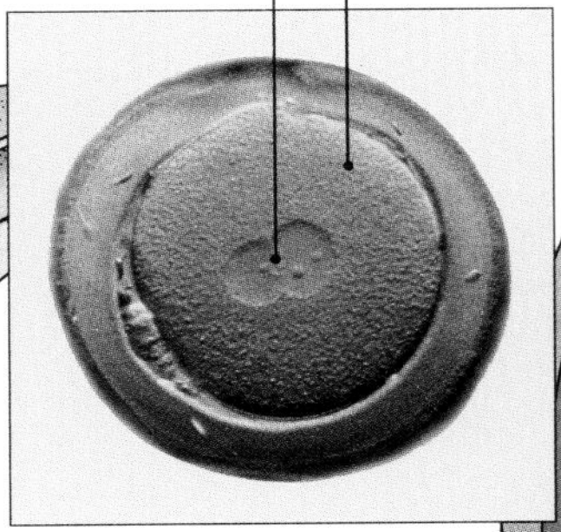

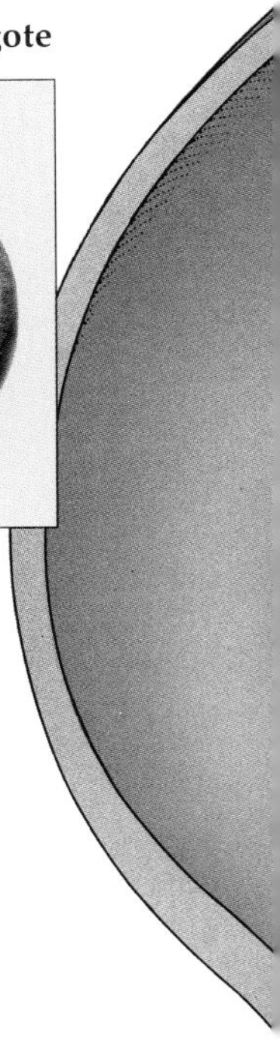

3 Sperm that reach the egg secrete an enzyme that breaks down the outer covering of the egg. Once a single sperm penetrates the egg, the chemical composition of the egg's outer covering rapidly changes, preventing other sperm from penetrating.

Fallopian tube

Fused nuclei   **Zygote**

Egg

Ovary

4 After the sperm has penetrated the egg, its tail separates from the head. The nucleus in the head of the sperm and the nucleus of the egg fuse, forming a fertilized egg. The fertilized egg is called a zygote.

Sperm

Uterus

INHERITANCE OF GENES

At the moment of fertilization, a unique set of genes is created – half from the man's sperm and half from the woman's egg. Genes are contained in paired structures called chromosomes. The fertilized egg acquires a total of 46 chromosomes – 23 pairs. The genes on the chromosomes – which will be present in every cell of the body of the fetus – carry all the inherited characteristics that determine how a person looks and how his or her body functions.

1 During sexual intercourse, 300 million or more sperm are ejaculated into the vagina. Only about 3 million of the sperm penetrate the cervix to reach the uterus; the rest are killed by the acidic secretions in the vagina or are lost through excretion from the woman's body.

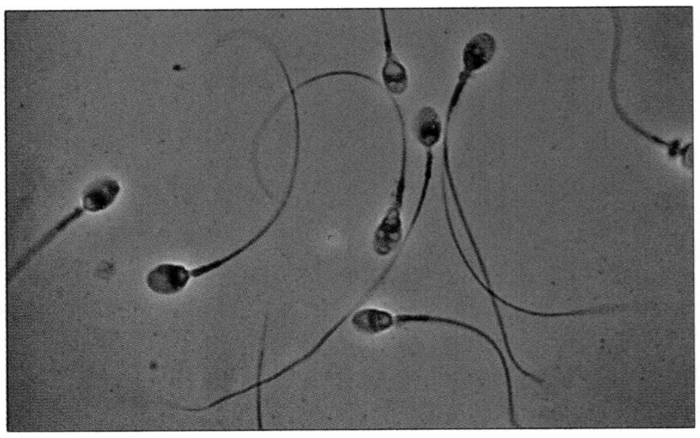

Cervix

Sperm

Vagina

The right place at the right time
Although some sperm (shown above, magnified 800 times) reach the fallopian tubes within half an hour of ejaculation, most sperm take about 4 to 7 hours. Sperm are capable of fertilization for 24 to 48 hours; an egg can be fertilized for 12 to 24 hours after release from the ovary (ovulation). Fertilization is most likely when sexual intercourse occurs between 2 days before and 1 day after ovulation.

FROM FERTILIZED EGG TO EMBRYO

Immediately after fertilization of the egg and before the egg becomes implanted in the endometrium (the lining of the uterus), an intricate series of events takes place as the fertilized egg moves down the fallopian tube toward the uterus.

2 The cells of the zygote continue to divide rapidly. Three to 4 days after fertilization, the zygote has developed into a solid cluster of cells called a morula.

HOW ARE TWINS FORMED?

A fertilized egg sometimes divides into two zygotes, which results in identical twins. The twins will be of the same sex and will be genetically identical. If two eggs are released from the ovary and are fertilized by different sperm, fraternal (nonidentical) twins result. Nonidentical twins may be of the same sex or different sexes.

Zygote

Morula

1 Within 24 hours after fertilization, the fertilized egg (called a zygote) divides into two cells.

3 The cells of the morula continue to divide. The morula develops into a structure called a blastocyst. The blastocyst has a fluid-filled cavity with a cluster of cells at one end. This cluster of cells will form the embryo. The outer layer of cells of the blastocyst is called the trophoblast.

Cluster of cells

Blastocyst

Trophoblast

Fluid-filled cavity

Cluster of cells

Trophoblast

HOW IS SEX DETERMINED?

The sex of a fetus is determined by a single pair of chromosomes called the sex chromosomes. Females have two almost identical sex chromosomes called X chromosomes. Males have one X chromosome and a smaller one called a Y chromosome.

A girl or a boy?
The sperm and egg each carry half of the pair of sex chromosomes. Each sperm has an X or a Y chromosome. Each egg has an X chromosome. If an egg is fertilized by a sperm with an X chromosome, the fetus will have two X chromosomes – a female. If an egg is fertilized by a sperm with a Y chromosome, the fetus will have one X and one Y chromosome – a male.

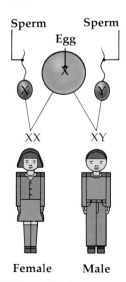

Sperm **Sperm**

Egg

X   Y

XX   XY

Female   **Male**

Endometrium

4 Five to 8 days after fertilization, the blastocyst attaches itself to the endometrium. The cells of the trophoblast layer penetrate the endometrium and spread around the implanted cluster of cells (the developing embryo). The trophoblast will form the placenta and the membranes that surround the embryo.

PLANNING FOR PREGNANCY

To give your baby the best possible start in life, you and your partner should begin planning for pregnancy at least 3 months before you conceive. You can take several steps that will increase your chances of conception and also be your best guarantee of having a healthy baby.

Deciding to have a baby is one of the most important decisions you will ever make. You and your partner should talk about, plan for, and learn all about pregnancy, the process of labor and childbirth, and parenting. You also need to carefully consider the changes and responsibilities that parenthood will bring to both of your lives. Talk to your doctor about your medical history to evaluate possible risks during pregnancy.

DECIDING TO HAVE A BABY

Before you decide to become pregnant, consider any possible risks and think about the effect that a baby will have on your lifestyle, your finances, and your career.

What effect will having a baby have on your finances?
Having a baby is expensive. You and your partner will want to discuss the financial adjustments you will need to make after the baby is born and the effects these adjustments will have on your life-style.

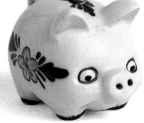

What about your age?
Pregnancy at any age carries some risks. Although medical advances have greatly reduced these risks, there is a gradual increase in your chance of having a baby with an abnormality as you get older (see page 20). Yet your general health, level of physical fitness, and medical history are much more important than age in influencing the health of your baby.

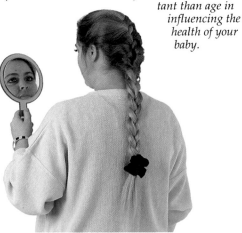

What effect will parenthood have on your career?
There may be times in your career when it is easier to take time off to have and/or raise a child. You and your partner should discuss the effect that having a baby will have on your career. Will you quit your job or return to work after the baby is born? Find out your company's policy on maternity leave and check into the types of childcare that are available.

What is your partner's attitude?
Having a baby brings many hopes and joys as well as concerns and fears to both partners. Talk to your partner about your feelings and the responsibilities of parenthood. Understanding, support, and reassurance are very important, both during your pregnancy and after your baby is born.

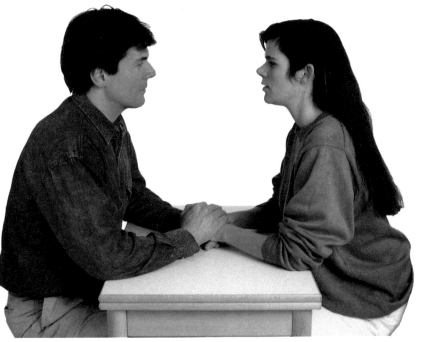

ASSESS YOUR HEALTH

Before you become pregnant, evaluate your health habits. A healthy life-style will improve your chances of conceiving, help reduce any risks during your pregnancy, and give your baby the strongest possible start in life.

Diet and fitness

If you are planning to have a baby, healthy eating habits and regular exercise are extremely important. Eat a well-balanced diet and drink six to eight glasses of liquids every day. Avoid foods that are high in fat, cholesterol, sugar, and sodium. Try to get your weight into the recommended range before you become pregnant. Being overweight increases your chances of developing high blood pressure during pregnancy, especially if you are over 35.

Talk to your doctor about including vitamin and mineral supplements in your diet. A folic acid supplement (see below) is recommended for women who are at high risk of having a child with a neural tube defect (a developmental failure of the brain and spinal cord).

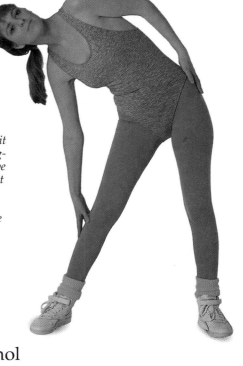

Getting in shape
Women who are healthy and in good physical condition have fewer problems during their pregnancies. Get as physically fit as you can before becoming pregnant. If you don't currently have a regular exercise program, start with a modest level of exercise (such as swimming or brisk walking) and gradually increase the time you spend exercising.

Smoking and alcohol

Smoking reduces fertility in both men and women, possibly by causing damage to eggs or by reducing the ability of sperm to penetrate an egg. Smoking during pregnancy can slow the growth of the fetus and raise your risk of miscarriage or stillbirth. Cigarette smoke affects blood flow to the placenta, causing babies of women who smoke (or who live with someone who smokes) to tend to have low birth weights. Babies with low birth weights frequently have serious health problems early in life.

Consuming alcohol during pregnancy increases the risk of miscarriage, stillbirth, and death in early infancy. Drinking excessive amounts of alcohol during pregnancy – or even a single binge shortly after conception – can result in the baby being born with fetal alcohol syndrome (physical and mental abnormalities).

No alcohol
To avoid any possible risk to the developing fetus, you should stop drinking alcohol once you decide to try to become pregnant and abstain from drinking alcohol throughout your pregnancy.

Folic acid
Doctors recommend that women who are at high risk of having a baby with a neural tube defect (such as spina bifida) take folic acid before conception and throughout the first 3 months of pregnancy. Couples who are in this high-risk group are those who have a neural tube defect themselves, who have had a child with a neural tube defect, or who have a close relative with such a condition.

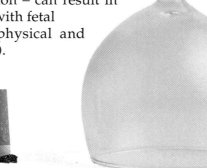

Stop smoking
If you are planning to become pregnant, stop smoking. Urge your partner to stop too.

EVALUATE POSSIBLE RISKS

In addition to adopting a healthy lifestyle, you should discuss possible risk factors in your medical history with your doctor before trying to become pregnant.

Effect of age

Although a woman over 35 may have difficulty conceiving, her chances of having a healthy baby do not differ significantly from those of a younger woman if she follows the basic health recommendations for pregnancy. However, women over 35 have a greater risk of bearing a child with certain birth defects, particularly Down's syndrome

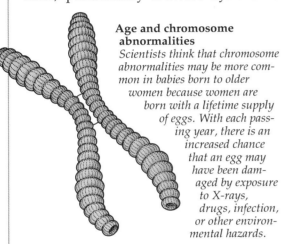

Age and chromosome abnormalities
Scientists think that chromosome abnormalities may be more common in babies born to older women because women are born with a lifetime supply of eggs. With each passing year, there is an increased chance that an egg may have been damaged by exposure to X-rays, drugs, infection, or other environmental hazards.

(a combination of mental retardation and physical abnormalities caused by the presence of an extra chromosome). Women over 35 also have an increased risk of miscarriage during the first trimester of the pregnancy.

Medical conditions

Some medical conditions, such as diabetes, high blood pressure, and asthma, can be dangerous to both the woman and the developing fetus. To reduce any possible risks caused by such conditions, early and regular monitoring of your pregnancy is essential. Talk to your doctor about any medical conditions you have before you try to conceive. Your doctor can advise you about special care

More older women are having babies
The large number of women born during the baby boom and the trend among many women to delay childbearing have contributed to the increased number of older women giving birth. It has been estimated that the total number of births among women 35 to 49 years old will increase from about 5 percent in 1982 to almost 9 percent by the year 2000.

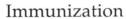

you will need during pregnancy. Also talk to your doctor about the possible effects that any medications you are taking could have on a fetus.

Immunization

Rubella (German measles) infection in early pregnancy can cause serious birth defects. Before you conceive, ask your doctor to verify that you are immune to rubella. If you are not immune, your doctor can vaccinate you against the infection. After getting the vaccination, you should wait at least 3 months – until immunity develops – before trying to become pregnant.

Doctors recommend that all pregnant women be tested for hepatitis B virus infection. If you are in a high-risk group for hepatitis, your doctor may recommend that you be vaccinated before trying to become pregnant.

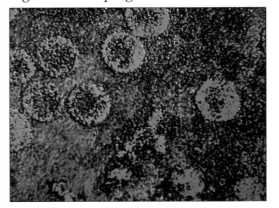

Hepatitis B virus
The hepatitis B virus (shown left, magnified 400,000 times) – one of the viruses that causes hepatitis (inflammation of the liver) – may be passed from an infected woman to her fetus during pregnancy or to her baby during delivery.

HIV AND AIDS

If you think you may have been exposed to the human immunodeficiency virus (HIV, the virus that causes AIDS), talk to your doctor before you become pregnant. A pregnant woman infected with HIV can pass the virus to her fetus. The rate of transmission during pregnancy ranges from 25 to 50 percent.

Genetic disorders

If you or your partner has a genetic (inherited) disorder, if there is a family history of genetic disorders, or if you have had a child with a genetic disorder, you may wish to talk to a genetic counselor before you decide to conceive. For some genetic disorders, tests are available to detect a defective gene. Along with the inheritance patterns for genetic disorders described below, genetic disorders can be passed to a fetus on one defective, so-called dominant gene. A parent who has the dominant gene has the disorder. Each child of an affected parent has a 1 in 2 chance of having the disorder.

WHAT IS A CARRIER?

A carrier of a genetic disorder has a gene for the disorder but is unaffected by it. The carrier can transmit the disorder to his or her offspring in one of two ways.

Recessive inheritance
A recessive genetic disorder occurs only when a child inherits two defective genes (one from each parent). Usually both parents are unaffected carriers of the defective gene. Each of their children has a 1 in 4 chance of being affected by the disorder and a 1 in 2 chance of being a carrier.

X-linked inheritance
X-linked genetic disorders are caused by defects on the X sex chromosome. A woman with a defect on one X chromosome is not affected because the defect is masked by her other, normal X chromosome, but a male who inherits the defective X chromosome will be affected. If a woman carries this defective gene, each son has a 1 in 2 chance of being affected; each daughter has a 1 in 2 chance of being a carrier.

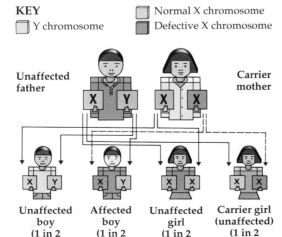

KEY ☐ Normal gene ■ Defective gene

Carrier father (unaffected) — Carrier mother (unaffected)

Unaffected child (1 in 4 chance) | Carrier child (unaffected) (1 in 2 chance) | Carrier child (unaffected) (1 in 2 chance) | Affected child (1 in 4 chance)

KEY ☐ Y chromosome ☐ Normal X chromosome ■ Defective X chromosome

Unaffected father — Carrier mother

Unaffected boy (1 in 2 chance) | Affected boy (1 in 2 chance) | Unaffected girl (1 in 2 chance) | Carrier girl (unaffected) (1 in 2 chance)

ASK YOUR DOCTOR
BECOMING PREGNANT

Q I have three sons and would like to have a girl next time. Is there anything I can do to influence the sex of my next baby?

A No. For centuries people have circulated claims that the sex of a child could be influenced by diet, the timing and frequency of intercourse, or the positions used for intercourse. There is no evidence to support these claims. The sex of the baby is determined at conception by a pair of chromosomes – one from the woman and one from the man.

Q Is it true that a woman is more likely to get pregnant if she lies still for a while after intercourse? And does a woman need to have an orgasm in order to conceive?

A The likelihood of becoming pregnant is not increased in any way by the woman lying still after intercourse. A few minutes after ejaculation, the healthiest sperm are deep inside a woman's body. Having an orgasm has no influence on a woman's chances of conceiving.

Q My husband and I are thinking about starting a family. A year ago I was diagnosed as having the viral infection genital herpes. What are the chances of passing this infection to the fetus?

A Passing genital herpes infection to the fetus is rare. Although the infection can be passed from an infected woman to her baby during vaginal delivery, in many cases this transmission can be prevented. If you have an active infection when you are about to deliver your baby, a cesarean section will be performed.

CONCEPTION

Men and women both become fertile (able to reproduce) at puberty. Men remain fertile well into old age; women remain fertile until the menopause. A couple at the peak age of fertility (in their 20s) – using no contraception and having intercourse regularly (at least once or twice a week) – has a 1 in 4 or 5 chance of conceiving in each menstrual cycle. The likelihood of conception decreases with age. Most women are unlikely to become pregnant the first month after they stop using contraception, but the majority are able to conceive within a few months.

Effect of contraceptive use

Most forms of birth control do not affect your ability to conceive once you stop using them. However, an intrauterine device (IUD) can lead to complications that affect fertility. IUDs increase the risk of pelvic inflammatory disease (severe or recurrent pelvic infection), which can cause infertility. If you have used an IUD and are unable to become pregnant after

6 months, see your doctor. If you have been taking birth control pills, your doctor may recommend that you stop taking them at least 3 months before you try to become pregnant. This interval will allow your usual menstrual cycle to resume, making it easier to pinpoint the time of ovulation.

Optimum time for conception

The most likely time for conception is 2 days before and 1 day after ovulation. To determine when you are ovulating, you can use a kit to test the level of luteinizing hormone in your urine (which increases just before ovulation) or the two methods shown below.

INCREASING YOUR CHANCES OF CONCEPTION

Sperm are best produced and stored when the temperature of the testicles is cooler than body temperature. A couple's chances of conception may be increased if the man wears loose-fitting underwear and pants (which keeps the testicles away from the body's heat) and does not take a hot bath just before sexual intercourse.

Cervical mucus method
To determine when you are ovulating, examine your vaginal secretions every day. Chart the changes in quantity, appearance, and texture of the mucus. Before ovulation, the mucus is sticky and breaks easily when stretched between your fingers. The amount of mucus increases almost 20-fold just before and for about 3 days after ovulation and the mucus becomes slippery and stretches more easily.

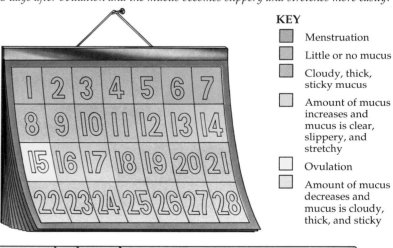

KEY

- Menstruation
- Little or no mucus
- Cloudy, thick, sticky mucus
- Amount of mucus increases and mucus is clear, slippery, and stretchy
- Ovulation
- Amount of mucus decreases and mucus is cloudy, thick, and sticky

Temperature method
To determine the time of ovulation, take your temperature before you get out of bed each morning and record it on a chart. Use a basal body thermometer, which is marked in fractions of degrees. For most women, body temperature increases slightly immediately after ovulation and stays at this level until just before menstruation. Typical temperature changes during the menstrual cycle are shown below.

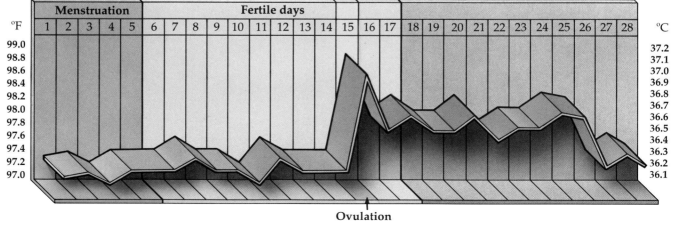

CASE HISTORY
DIFFICULTY CONCEIVING

S COTT AND JENNIFER **had been trying for more than a year to start a family, but Jennifer had not become pregnant. Since Jennifer had stopped using birth control pills more than 1 ½ years ago, she and Scott became worried that something was wrong. Jennifer made an appointment to see her gynecologist.**

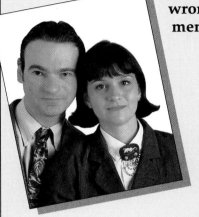

PERSONAL DETAILS
Names Scott and Jennifer Lewis
Ages Scott is 33; Jennifer is 32
Occupations Scott is a stockbroker; Jennifer is an advertising executive
Family Scott's parents are in good health. Jennifer's mother is healthy; her father died of a heart attack last year.

MEDICAL BACKGROUND
Scott and Jennifer have not had any serious health problems. Jennifer's menstrual periods are regular. She has seen her gynecologist regularly for pelvic examinations and Pap smears, which have been normal.

THE CONSULTATION
Jennifer explains her concerns to her gynecologist. The doctor performs a physical and a pelvic examination. He tells her that he does not see anything wrong, but explains that infertility is a problem that often involves both partners. He recommends that Scott be examined by his doctor, and that Jennifer and Scott come to the office together.

The gynecologist is pleased to find out that Scott's checkup was normal. He asks Jennifer and Scott detailed questions about their medical histories and life-styles. He discovers that they both smoke and drink, rarely eat a well-balanced meal, and do not exercise regularly. Most important,

because both of their jobs involve a lot of traveling, Jennifer and Scott seldom have time together to have sexual intercourse.

THE DIAGNOSIS
The doctor suspects that Scott and Jennifer's infertility may be the result of their UNHEALTHY LIFE-STYLES AND INFREQUENT INTERCOURSE rather than any medical problems.

THE ADVICE
The gynecologist recommends that Scott and Jennifer quit smoking, stop drinking alcohol, eat a balanced diet, and start exercising regularly. The doctor explains to Jennifer how to take and record her daily temperature and note descriptions of her vaginal secretions to help determine when she is ovulating. The few days before and after ovulation are when she is most likely to conceive.

Jennifer and Scott return to the gynecologist a month later. They tell him that they both feel much

healthier now that they are following his recommendations. Jennifer tells the doctor that she discovered that her temperature rises on day 14 of her menstrual cycle and that her vaginal secretions change in consistency around this time too. The doctor explains to them that they have the best chance of conception if they have sexual intercourse around day 13 of Jennifer's menstrual cycle. He recommends that they make having sex at the right time each month a priority in their schedules.

THE OUTCOME
Four months later, Jennifer determines she is pregnant. She and Scott are both delighted and start making plans for the arrival of their baby.

Getting fit
Jennifer and Scott make an effort to eat better and they decide to walk, rather than drive, to work. They both quit smoking. Jennifer stops drinking alcohol; Scott has an occasional glass of wine.

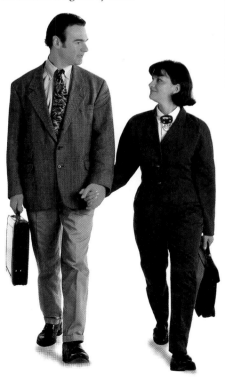

CHAPTER TWO

A HEALTHY PREGNANCY

INTRODUCTION

CONFIRMING
YOUR PREGNANCY

THE GROWING
FETUS

YOUR CHANGING
BODY

NO MATTER HOW MUCH planning they have done in preparation for starting a family, nearly all couples experience mixed feelings when the woman becomes pregnant. The discovery that they are bringing a new person into the world can be unsettling. While feeling great joy, the parents-to-be may also be concerned about the health of the baby, their ability to be good parents, their financial situation, and the impact a baby will have on their relationship. These feelings are normal. You and your partner need to share your feelings to help you both understand and deal with each other's concerns. Communication will help you relax, enjoy the experience of expectant parenthood, and celebrate the start of a new life.

A woman may worry about the physical changes her body will be undergoing, especially if this is her first pregnancy. Understanding how and

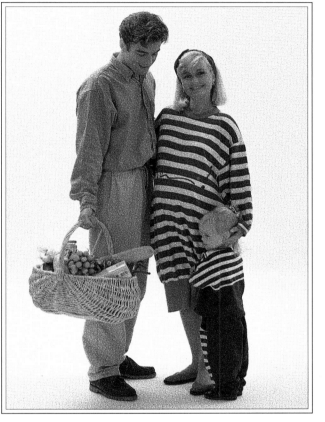

why your body undergoes certain changes will help relieve any anxieties you may have. Take a prenatal class, read books on pregnancy, and talk to your doctor so that you know what to expect. Prenatal care should be started as early as possible in your pregnancy so that potential problems can be identified and treated if necessary. Although in previous times pregnancy was a high-risk condition, most pregnancies today proceed naturally and normally. Your pregnancy is a unique, personal experience. No two women are identical, and each pregnancy develops differently, with milestones occurring at different times. Do not be alarmed if you have not experienced certain symptoms or changes that are discussed in this chapter. Most women feel healthy during pregnancy, and any unpleasant symptoms usually disappear by about the 12th week of the pregnancy.

This chapter tells you the signs that indicate you might be pregnant and explains the tests that you and your doctor may use to confirm your pregnancy. We explain two methods that you can use to estimate the delivery date of your baby. We give sensible advice and reassurance about what to expect in the early stages of your pregnancy. While the fetus is growing inside you, it is undergoing miraculous changes. We explain how the fetus develops and how your body will change and prepare for birth. The final section in the chapter discusses many of the symptoms and conditions that are commonly experienced by women during pregnancy and gives helpful tips that may help relieve some of the temporary discomfort. We also alert you to the warning signs of some problems that require immediate medical attention.

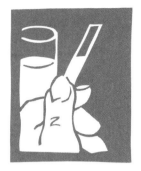

CONFIRMING YOUR PREGNANCY

SOME WOMEN seem to know when they become pregnant – they feel "different." This feeling of being pregnant before any physical signs are present may be the result of the secretion of hormones early in pregnancy. These hormones not only cause physical changes in your body, but can also affect emotions.

A missed period or unusual tenderness and fullness of your breasts is often the first physical sign that you are pregnant. Other early signs that you might be pregnant are nausea and vomiting, fatigue, and a frequent need to urinate. Every woman is different and may experience any or all of these signs. As soon as you suspect that you might be pregnant, you should see your doctor for confirmation (see PREGNANCY TESTS on page 28).

EARLY SIGNS OF PREGNANCY

Even before you have missed a menstrual period, you may notice changes in your breasts. Your breasts may feel full and tender, with tingling and soreness of the nipples. Increased production of the hormone progesterone produces these changes in the breasts. Other early signs of pregnancy that you may experience are explained in the illustration at right.

Morning sickness
Some research suggests that the body's production of the hormone human chorionic gonadotropin during pregnancy may stimulate the part of the brain that controls nausea and vomiting, causing so-called morning sickness. Morning sickness (not always confined to the morning) usually begins at about the sixth week of pregnancy (see HOW TO EASE MORNING SICKNESS on page 27).

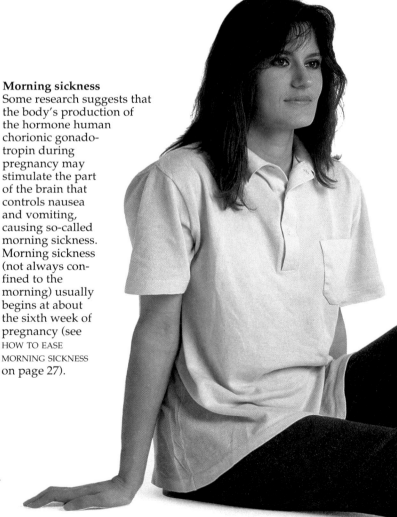

BREAST BEFORE PREGNANCY   BREAST DURING PREGNANCY

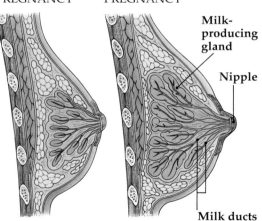

Milk-producing gland

Nipple

Milk ducts

Changes in the breasts
Your breasts will become larger because the glands and ducts inside them are preparing for nursing the baby when he or she is born. Your nipples become more prominent and darker; the veins near the surface of the breasts become more noticeable.

HOW TO EASE MORNING SICKNESS

One third to half of pregnant women experience morning sickness. The following tips may help relieve the symptoms.

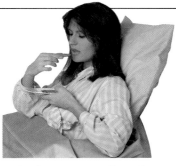

◆ Drink plenty of liquids, such as vegetable and fruit juices, milk, soups, and broth.

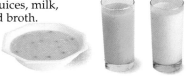

◆ Try to get some extra sleep and avoid stress.

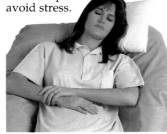

◆ Eat frequent, small meals. An empty stomach can trigger nausea. A high-protein snack, eaten at bedtime or first thing in the morning before you get up, may help minimize nausea and vomiting.

◆ Let plenty of fresh air into the house to eliminate food and household odors.

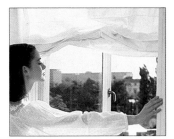

◆ Avoid greasy or spicy foods. Eat plenty of fruit and foods high in protein, such as lean meat and fish, and complex carbohydrates (starch and fiber), such as vegetables and whole-grain products.

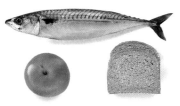

Tiredness
For some women, the first indication of pregnancy is being very tired. This fatigue may be caused by high levels of the hormone progesterone that are produced during pregnancy. Progesterone acts as a powerful, but natural, sedative and tranquilizer.

Missed period
A missed menstrual period is often the first sign of pregnancy. Sometimes, light bleeding may occur as a result of the implantation of the fertilized egg in the wall of the uterus.

Frequent need to urinate
As a result of the increased activity of hormones and the pressure of the enlarging uterus on the bladder during pregnancy, many women need to urinate much more frequently than usual. This symptom can begin as early as 1 week after conception.

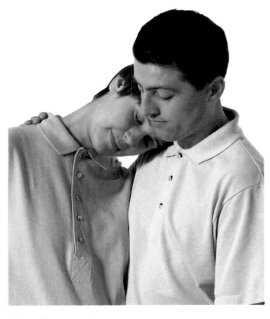

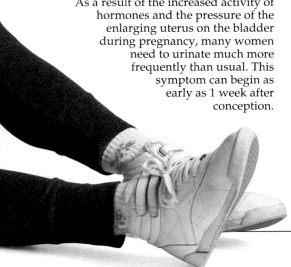

Changing emotions
Early in your pregnancy, you may experience many changes in your emotions – pleasure because you want a baby, anxiety about the baby's health, or concern about the responsibility of raising a child. You may be weepy one day and overjoyed the next. Some of these emotions are a normal – and temporary – response to your body's changing hormone levels. Support and understanding are important; talk to your partner about what you are feeling – he may be experiencing some of the same concerns.

CAUSES OF A MISSED PERIOD

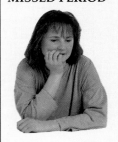

Pregnancy is not the only possible cause of a missed menstrual period. A late or missed period can be caused by anxiety, depression, stress, emotional shock, some medications, anorexia nervosa (an eating disorder), illness, surgery, or jet lag.

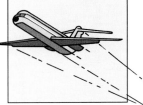

PREGNANCY TESTS

Three tests are most often used to confirm a pregnancy – all of which involve the detection of a hormone called human chorionic gonadotropin (HCG) in the urine or blood. In the early stages of pregnancy the growing placenta produces large quantities of HCG. HCG stimulates the ovaries to produce estrogen and progesterone, hormones needed to retain the endometrium (the lining of the uterus) in which the embryo grows and is nourished. The levels of HCG begin to diminish after week 12 as the placenta develops and becomes capable of producing the hormones necessary for growth and development of the fetus.

If you think that you might be pregnant, you can buy a kit to test your urine at home. Home pregnancy testing kits can detect HCG as early as the first day of a missed menstrual period (possibly 14 days after conception). If the result of your testing is positive, you should see your doctor as soon as possible to confirm the results. You may get a negative test result even though you are pregnant if the test is performed incorrectly or if you don't use a first-of-the-morning urine sample.

You may prefer to have your doctor perform the initial pregnancy test. Your doctor will send a sample of your urine to a laboratory, where methods similar to those in home testing kits are used. Home testing kits have a small error rate, but the accuracy of laboratory testing is nearly 100 percent, and a pregnancy can be confirmed 7 to 10 days after conception.

The third type of pregnancy test is a blood test to detect HCG. This test is the most reliable and can confirm a pregnancy 8 to 10 days after conception.

Blood test
A blood test to detect HCG is a routine test – and the most accurate test – for confirming pregnancy. The doctor may also test your blood to see if you are anemic, to check for syphilis, to see if you have had German measles, and to learn your blood type and Rh factor (see BLOOD TESTS on page 55). Repeated blood tests can help evaluate a suspected ectopic pregnancy (see page 86) or abnormalities during pregnancy.

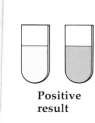

Negative result   Positive result

Home pregnancy testing kit
You can purchase several different types of home pregnancy testing kits. Most kits include a chemically coated stick that you dip into a first-of-the-morning sample of urine. Any change in color on the stick indicates a positive result.

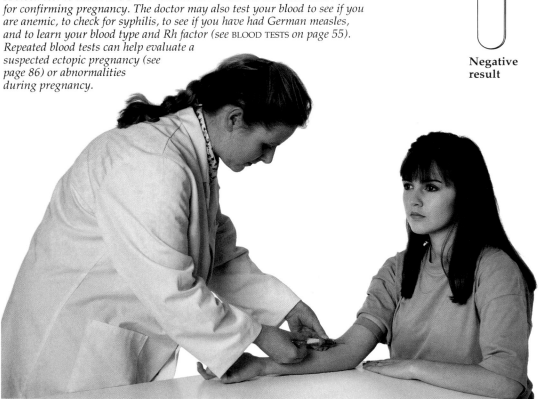

OTHER TESTS TO CONFIRM YOUR PREGNANCY

An internal examination (called a pelvic examination) is a routine part of your first visit to confirm your pregnancy (see page 53). In some cases, an ultrasound scan may be needed.

Pelvic examination
A pelvic examination helps your doctor determine the size of and changes in the uterus and the amount of room in your pelvis for the fetus. The doctor inserts two fingers into the vagina and gently pushes on the abdomen with his or her other hand.

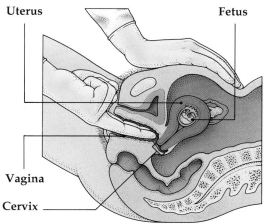

Uterus

Fetus

Vagina

Cervix

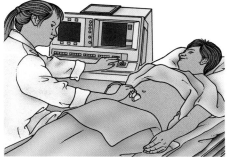

Ultrasound scanning
Ultrasound scanning (see page 58) is not a routine test to confirm a pregnancy. It is done if results of previous tests to confirm the pregnancy are unclear or conflicting. Ultrasound may also be done in special circumstances, such as a suspected ectopic pregnancy (see page 86).

YOUR ESTIMATED DELIVERY DATE

The average length of a pregnancy, calculated from the first day of your last menstrual period, is 280 days (40 weeks). To estimate your delivery date, take the date of the first day of your last period, add 7, then count back 3 months. For example, if your last period began on June 11th, add 7 to 11. Count back 3 months. Your estimated delivery date will be March 18th. This method is based on a 28-day menstrual cycle. If your menstrual cycle is longer than 28 days, you are likely to deliver after this date; if your cycle is shorter, you may deliver before this date (the chart below uses a slightly different method). Few babies arrive exactly on their estimated date of delivery. It is normal for a pregnancy to last between 37 and 42 weeks.

An ultrasound scan (see page 58) is sometimes used to estimate a delivery date for women who are unsure of the date of their last period or who may have an irregular menstrual cycle.

Estimated delivery dates
The chart at left gives calculations of delivery dates that are based on counting forward 40 weeks from the first day of your last menstrual period. Find the date of the first day of your last menstrual period in the lines of dates in bold type. The date directly below this number is your estimated delivery date.

Month	1	2	3	4	5	6	7	8	9	10	11	12	13	14	15	16	17	18	19	20	21	22	23	24	25	26	27	28	29	30	31
Jan Oct/Nov	8	9	10	11	12	13	14	15	16	17	18	19	20	21	22	23	24	25	26	27	28	29	30	31	1	2	3	4	5	6	7
Feb Nov/Dec	8	9	10	11	12	13	14	15	16	17	18	19	20	21	22	23	24	25	26	27	28	29	30	1	2	3	4	5			
Mar Dec/Jan	6	7	8	9	10	11	12	13	14	15	16	17	18	19	20	21	22	23	24	25	26	27	28	29	30	31	1	2	3	4	5
April Jan/Feb	6	7	8	9	10	11	12	13	14	15	16	17	18	19	20	21	22	23	24	25	26	27	28	29	30	31	1	2	3	4	
May Feb/Mar	5	6	7	8	9	10	11	12	13	14	15	16	17	18	19	20	21	22	23	24	25	26	27	28	1	2	3	4	5	6	7
June Mar/Apr	8	9	10	11	12	13	14	15	16	17	18	19	20	21	22	23	24	25	26	27	28	29	30	31	1	2	3	4	5	6	
July Apr/May	7	8	9	10	11	12	13	14	15	16	17	18	19	20	21	22	23	24	25	26	27	28	29	30	1	2	3	4	5	6	7
Aug May/June	8	9	10	11	12	13	14	15	16	17	18	19	20	21	22	23	24	25	26	27	28	29	30	31	1	2	3	4	5	6	7
Sept June/July	8	9	10	11	12	13	14	15	16	17	18	19	20	21	22	23	24	25	26	27	28	29	30	1	2	3	4	5	6	7	
Oct July/Aug	8	9	10	11	12	13	14	15	16	17	18	19	20	21	22	23	24	25	26	27	28	29	30	31	1	2	3	4	5	6	7
Nov Aug/Sept	8	9	10	11	12	13	14	15	16	17	18	19	20	21	22	23	24	25	26	27	28	29	30	31	1	2	3	4	5	6	
Dec Sept/Oct	7	8	9	10	11	12	13	14	15	16	17	18	19	20	21	22	23	24	25	26	27	28	29	30	1	2	3	4	5	6	7

THE GROWING FETUS

FETAL DEVELOPMENT is divided into three stages (called trimesters) of about 13 weeks each. By the end of the first trimester, the fetus's major organs have developed. During the second trimester, the fetus grows rapidly and you start to feel its first movements. During the third trimester, the fetus continues to grow and gains weight. From conception until the eighth week of pregnancy, the fertilized egg is called an embryo. From 8 weeks until birth, it is called a fetus.

IMPLANTATION

After fertilization, the egg begins to divide into a mass of cells (see FERTILIZATION OF AN EGG on page 16). Between 5 and 8 days after fertilization, this mass of cells (called a blastocyst) implants itself in the lining of the uterus. The blastocyst has an inner cluster of cells that will form the embryo and an outer layer known as the trophoblast.

2 WEEKS

Some cells of the trophoblast start to form the placenta; other cells of the trophoblast will form the membranes that surround the embryo (called the amniotic sac). The inner cluster of cells becomes organized into three separate layers – the ectoderm, mesoderm, and entoderm – that will form different parts of the embryo.

5 WEEKS

By the end of the fifth week, the basic human design has developed (see embryo below, magnified 4 ½ times). The arms and legs are forming. The eyes, nose, and mouth are starting to become visible. The umbilical cord has formed.

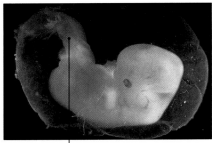

Umbilical cord

Entoderm

Cells that will form the amniotic sac

The layers that will form the embryo
The ectoderm (the outside layer of the cluster of cells within the blastocyst) will develop into the fetus's central nervous system, skin, hair, nails, tooth enamel, and parts of the sense organs (nose, ears, and eyes). The mesoderm (the middle layer) will develop into bone, muscle, cartilage, connective tissue, the heart, blood cells and blood vessels, and lymph cells and lymph vessels. The entoderm (the inside layer) will develop into the digestive tract, respiratory tract, bladder, tonsils, thyroid gland, liver, and pancreas, and the linings of the eardrums and eustachian tubes.

Ectoderm

Mesoderm

Placenta beginning to form

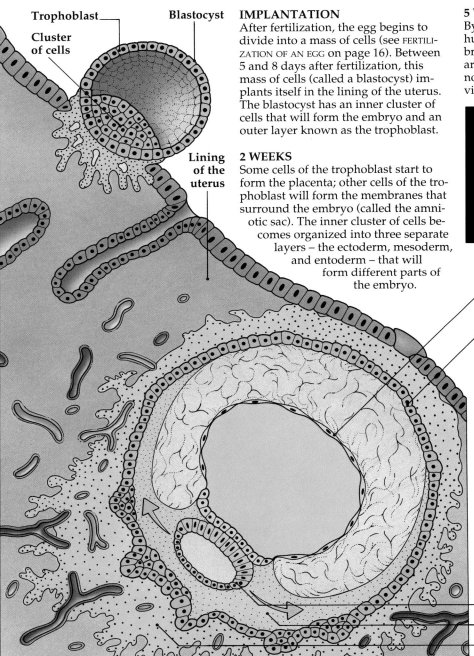

Trophoblast

Cluster of cells

Blastocyst

Lining of the uterus

THE FETUS'S LIFE-SUPPORT SYSTEM

While inside the uterus, the growing fetus receives nourishment from the placenta, to which it is linked by the umbilical cord. The fetus floats in the amniotic fluid, which is contained within a protective membrane called the amniotic sac. The placenta, umbilical cord, and amniotic fluid are vital parts of the fetus's system of life support.

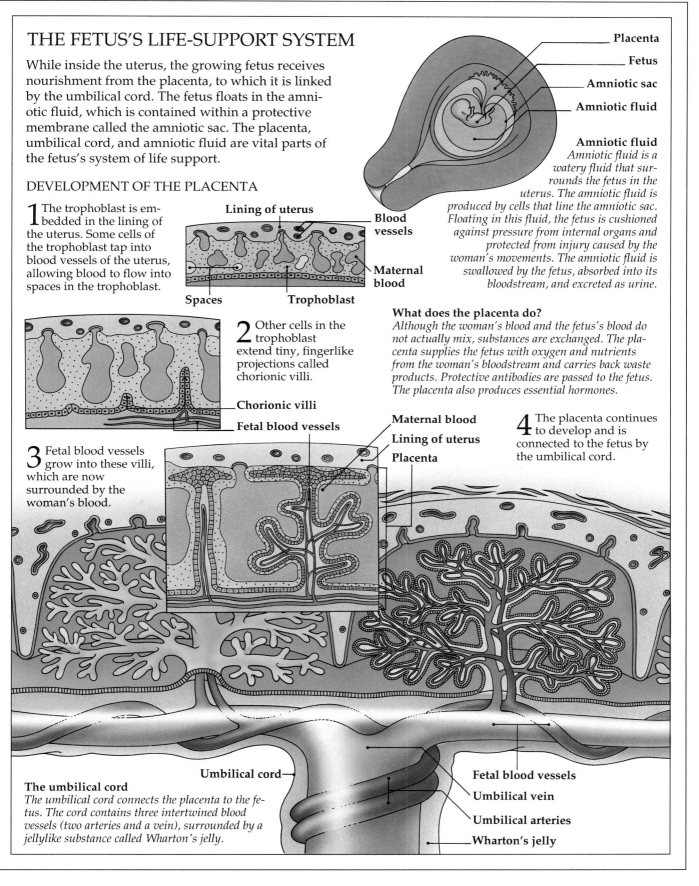

Placenta

Fetus

Amniotic sac

Amniotic fluid

DEVELOPMENT OF THE PLACENTA

1 The trophoblast is embedded in the lining of the uterus. Some cells of the trophoblast tap into blood vessels of the uterus, allowing blood to flow into spaces in the trophoblast.

Lining of uterus

Blood vessels

Maternal blood

Spaces

Trophoblast

Amniotic fluid
Amniotic fluid is a watery fluid that surrounds the fetus in the uterus. The amniotic fluid is produced by cells that line the amniotic sac. Floating in this fluid, the fetus is cushioned against pressure from internal organs and protected from injury caused by the woman's movements. The amniotic fluid is swallowed by the fetus, absorbed into its bloodstream, and excreted as urine.

2 Other cells in the trophoblast extend tiny, fingerlike projections called chorionic villi.

Chorionic villi

Fetal blood vessels

What does the placenta do?
Although the woman's blood and the fetus's blood do not actually mix, substances are exchanged. The placenta supplies the fetus with oxygen and nutrients from the woman's bloodstream and carries back waste products. Protective antibodies are passed to the fetus. The placenta also produces essential hormones.

3 Fetal blood vessels grow into these villi, which are now surrounded by the woman's blood.

Maternal blood

Lining of uterus

Placenta

4 The placenta continues to develop and is connected to the fetus by the umbilical cord.

Umbilical cord

The umbilical cord
The umbilical cord connects the placenta to the fetus. The cord contains three intertwined blood vessels (two arteries and a vein), surrounded by a jellylike substance called Wharton's jelly.

Fetal blood vessels

Umbilical vein

Umbilical arteries

Wharton's jelly

ACTUAL SIZE

Weeks

- 2
- 3
- 4
- 5
- 6

- 8

6 WEEKS
Length: ½ inch
The embryo's head is forming and the brain, spine, and nervous system are developing. There are four shallow depressions on its head that will later become the eyes and ears. The abdomen and digestive system begin to develop – the embryo now has primitive forms of a jaw, mouth, and stomach. The heart, still only a single tube, can be seen as a bulge at the front of the chest and will begin beating by the end of the sixth week. Muscles start to form, over which the skin begins to grow.

8 WEEKS
Length: 1 inch
The embryo is now called a fetus. All the major internal organs have formed. The arms and legs are clearly visible, with shoulders, elbows, hips, and knees. The fingers and toes are distinct, although they are still joined by webs of skin. Blood cells have developed and blood is circulating around the fetus's body in primitive blood vessels. The fetus's eyes, nose, and mouth are more recognizable. The ears are beginning to develop as buds on either side of the head. The fetus begins to move around.

8 WEEKS

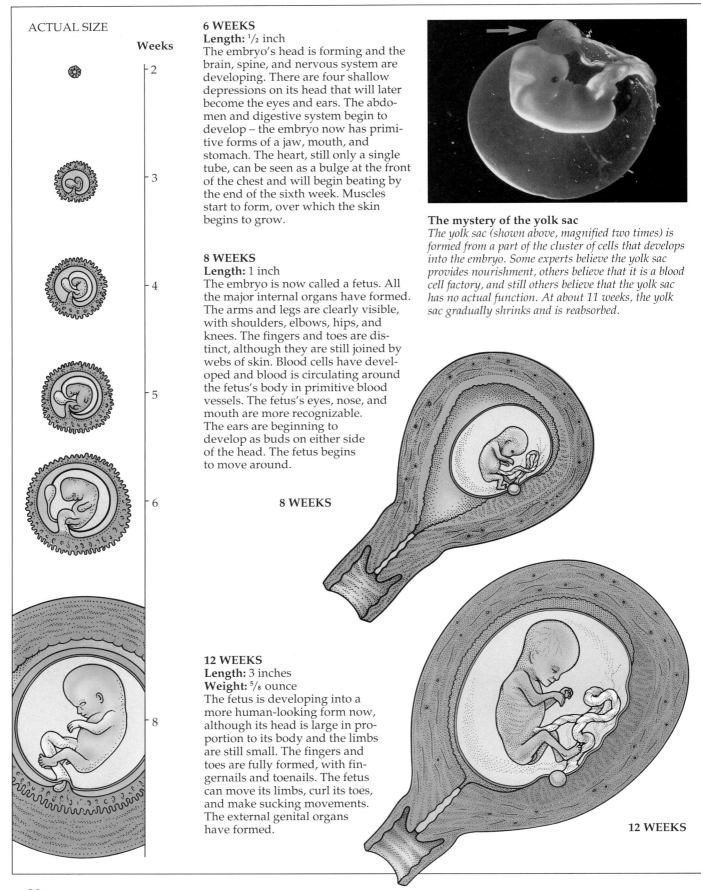

The mystery of the yolk sac
The yolk sac (shown above, magnified two times) is formed from a part of the cluster of cells that develops into the embryo. Some experts believe the yolk sac provides nourishment, others believe that it is a blood cell factory, and still others believe that the yolk sac has no actual function. At about 11 weeks, the yolk sac gradually shrinks and is reabsorbed.

12 WEEKS
Length: 3 inches
Weight: ⅝ ounce
The fetus is developing into a more human-looking form now, although its head is large in proportion to its body and the limbs are still small. The fingers and toes are fully formed, with fingernails and toenails. The fetus can move its limbs, curl its toes, and make sucking movements. The external genital organs have formed.

12 WEEKS

16 WEEKS
Length: 6 inches
Weight: 4 ³/₄ ounces
The fetus's limbs and joints are fully formed and the muscles are getting stronger. The fetus now even has its own unique fingerprints. Vigorous movements are taking place, although the woman does not always feel them at this early stage. During the rest of the pregnancy the fetus grows and the internal organs mature. Fine, downy hair (called lanugo hair) grows on the fetus's body and the eyelashes and eyebrows start to grow. The fetus's heartbeat can be heard with an ultrasound device.

16 WEEKS

20 WEEKS
Length: 10 inches
Weight: 12 ounces
The fetus is now growing rapidly and the arms and legs have grown into proportion with the rest of the body. The woman may now feel the fetus's movements as faint flutters inside her abdomen. Teeth are forming in the fetus's jawbone and hair is growing on its head.

24 WEEKS
Length: 13 inches
Weight: 1 ¹/₄ pounds
The fetus continues to grow rapidly, although it has not yet begun to store fat. The eyes appear to bulge from the face. The fetus is able to hiccup, cough, and suck its thumb.

32 WEEKS
Length: 16 inches
Weight: 3 ¹/₂ pounds
The head is now in the same proportion to the body as it will be at birth. The fetus begins to store fat. The fetus's body is covered in a waxy substance called vernix that protects the skin. In most cases, the fetus lies with its head down toward the pelvis. The woman can easily feel the fetus's vigorous movements.

36 WEEKS
Length: 18 inches
Weight: 5 ¹/₂ pounds
The fetus now fills the uterus, and the woman can feel its movements more forcefully. The head may have dropped down into the area of the pelvis in preparation for the birth. The fetus's body becomes more rounded as more fat is stored. The irises of the fetus's eyes are blue, and the hair on its head may be up to 2 inches long. The fetus's nails have grown to the end of the toes and fingers. In a male fetus, the testicles should have descended from inside the fetus's body.

40 WEEKS
Length: 20 inches
Weight: 7 ¹/₂ pounds
The fetus is now fully developed. When the fetus is awake, its eyes are open and it can discern light and dark. Most of the vernix has come off the body, remaining only in the skin folds around the neck, armpits, and groin. Most of the soft lanugo hair has disappeared.

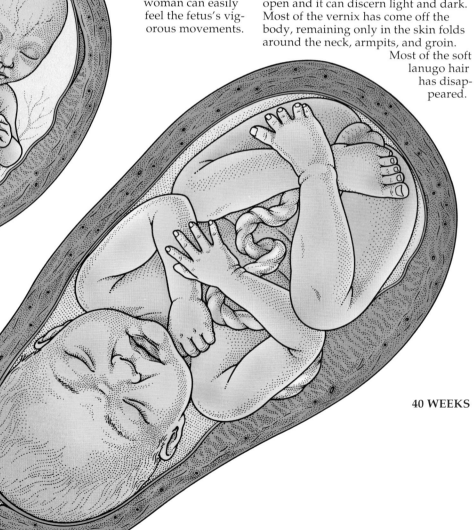

40 WEEKS

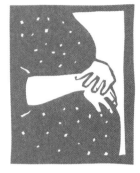

YOUR CHANGING BODY

URING THE 9 MONTHS OF PREGNANCY, the fetus develops from an embryo smaller than a grain of rice to an infant with an average birth weight of about 7 ½ pounds. A woman's body also undergoes many changes as it adapts to the growing fetus and prepares to give birth – every organ in her body is affected in some way. These changes may cause some temporary discomforts that are a natural and normal part of having a baby.

CHANGES IN YOUR CIRCULATION

Throughout pregnancy, changes take place in your circulatory system (your heart and blood vessels). The volume of blood that is being pumped by your heart increases by about 40 percent. To accommodate this increased volume of blood, your heart enlarges slightly, your heart rate rises from about 70 to 85 beats per minute, and the amount of blood that is pumped out with each heartbeat increases. Your blood pressure is lower because increased production of certain hormones during pregnancy causes blood vessels to widen. This widening of the vessels decreases their resistance to blood flow, lowering blood pressure.

Many of the changes in your body that occur during pregnancy are visible – the increase in the size of your breasts and abdomen, for example. Inside your body, other changes are taking place so that you can nourish and accommodate the growing fetus. Most of these are caused by fluctuations in hormone levels during pregnancy. It is important that you understand the changes in your body so that you can determine what is normal and what may require medical attention.

Blood flow
During the last trimester of your pregnancy, you may feel faint or dizzy when you get up after lying on your back. This feeling is caused by a reduced amount of blood being pumped to your brain. When you lie on your back, your uterus may press on the inferior vena cava (the large vein that returns blood to the heart from the lower parts of your body). The pressure on this vein reduces blood flow to the heart, which then pumps out less blood through the aorta to the rest of the body.

LYING ON YOUR BACK

Uterus

Aorta   Spine   Inferior vena cava

LYING ON YOUR SIDE

Spine

Aorta

Inferior vena cava

Uterus

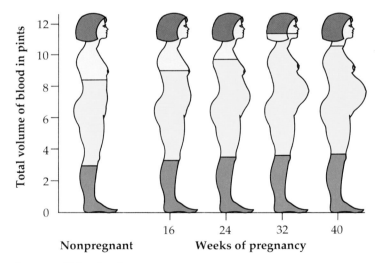

Nonpregnant   Weeks of pregnancy

Increased blood volume
The amount of blood in your body (called the blood volume) increases during pregnancy by at least 40 percent – about an extra 3 pints. The volume of plasma (the fluid part of blood) increases more than the volume of the red blood cells (see above). The increased amount of blood is required to supply the growing fetus with oxygen and nutrients as well as to meet the increased demands of your body. The blood volume decreases toward the end of pregnancy, which enables the woman to better tolerate the stress of labor and delivery.

KEY

 Plasma volume

 Red blood cell volume

THE ROLE OF HORMONES DURING PREGNANCY

Most of the changes that take place in your body while you are pregnant are stimulated by hormones.

Thyroid gland
During pregnancy, the thyroid gland increases its production of the hormones thyroxine and triiodothyronine. These hormones cause many of the body's tissues to increase their metabolic rates (the rates at which the tissues burn up oxygen and fuels such as fat, carbohydrate, and protein to produce energy). The increased rate of metabolism produces more body heat, causes increased blood flow to the skin to promote heat loss, and makes the heart work harder in order to meet the body's increased demand for oxygen.

Kidneys

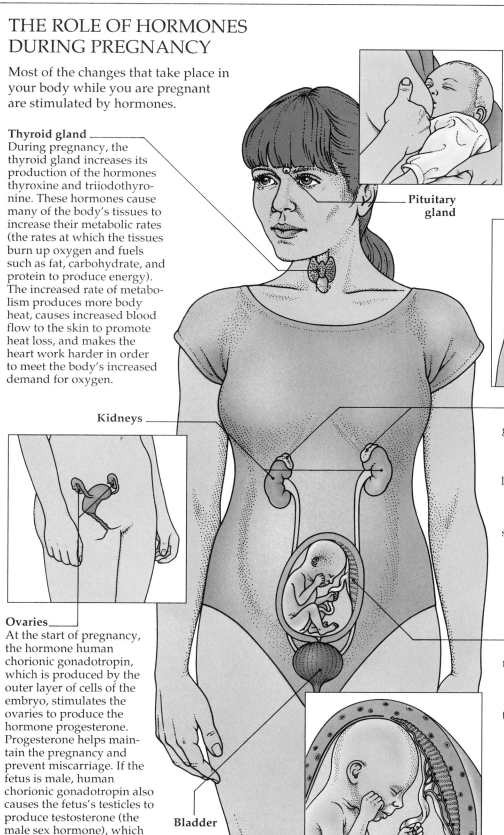

Pituitary gland

Bladder

Ovaries
At the start of pregnancy, the hormone human chorionic gonadotropin, which is produced by the outer layer of cells of the embryo, stimulates the ovaries to produce the hormone progesterone. Progesterone helps maintain the pregnancy and prevent miscarriage. If the fetus is male, human chorionic gonadotropin also causes the fetus's testicles to produce testosterone (the male sex hormone), which stimulates the development of the fetus's sex organs.

Pituitary gland
The hormone prolactin, produced by the pituitary gland during pregnancy, helps prepare your breast tissues for milk production. After your baby has been born, prolactin stimulates the production of milk; this effect is suppressed during your pregnancy by the high levels of estrogen being produced.

Adrenal glands
During pregnancy, the adrenal glands produce large quantities of corticosteroid hormones. These hormones regulate the body's use of nutrients, the levels of sodium and potassium in the blood, and the amounts of sodium and potassium excreted in the urine. Corticosteroid hormones also suppress inflammatory reactions, which may explain why inflammatory conditions such as rheumatoid arthritis often ease during pregnancy.

Placenta
The placenta produces hormones that stimulate growth of the uterus and breast tissue during pregnancy. When fully developed (at about 10 weeks), the placenta becomes the major site of production of the hormone progesterone, which was produced almost entirely by the ovaries earlier in the pregnancy. The placenta also produces the hormone human placental lactogen, which – along with prolactin – stimulates changes in your breast tissues in preparation for the production of milk.

35

BREATHING

During pregnancy, your lungs need to work harder to keep the increased volume of blood in your body supplied with oxygen. Your respiratory rate (the number of breaths you take per minute) does not usually change. Rather, the increased demands for oxygen are met by an increase in the volume of air you can inhale (see right).

Before pregnancy

During pregnancy

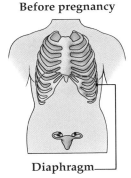
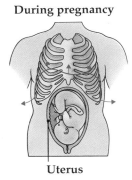

Diaphragm

Uterus

Taking larger breaths
As your uterus enlarges, your diaphragm is pushed upward about 2 inches and its range of movement increases by $1/2$ to 1 inch. The circumference of your chest also increases by 2 to 3 inches. These changes allow you to inhale a larger volume of air.

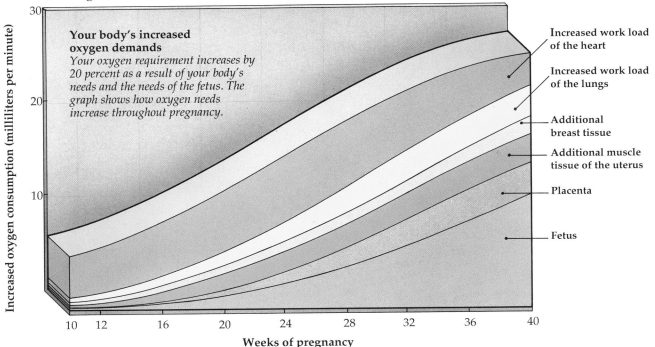

Your body's increased oxygen demands
Your oxygen requirement increases by 20 percent as a result of your body's needs and the needs of the fetus. The graph shows how oxygen needs increase throughout pregnancy.

Increased oxygen consumption (milliliters per minute)

Weeks of pregnancy

Increased work load of the heart

Increased work load of the lungs

Additional breast tissue

Additional muscle tissue of the uterus

Placenta

Fetus

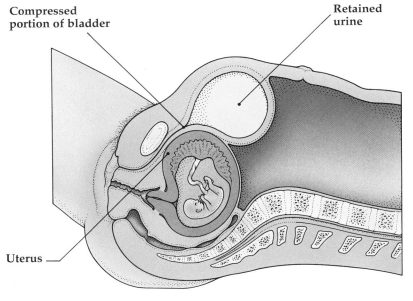

Compressed portion of bladder

Retained urine

Uterus

KIDNEYS AND BLADDER

Your kidneys filter your blood and excrete waste products and excess water in urine. When you are pregnant, your kidneys must filter a larger volume of blood. Consequently, they excrete a larger volume of waste products and water. You may feel thirsty, drink more liquids than usual, and urinate more often. Pressure of the growing uterus on your bladder may also increase the urge to urinate.

Retention of urine during pregnancy
In rare instances, the enlarging uterus compresses the bladder so that the bladder cannot be emptied completely. This retention of urine can result in an infection of the urinary tract.

DIGESTION

During pregnancy, an increased level of the hormone progesterone causes the muscles in the digestive tract to relax. Relaxation of the muscles at the lower end of the esophagus (the tube through which food passes from the throat to the stomach) may cause heartburn. As a result of the relaxation of muscles in the large intestine, passage of stools becomes less efficient, which can lead to constipation.

Heartburn

The relaxation of muscles at the junction of the esophagus and the stomach may allow food mixed with stomach acids to be pushed up from the stomach into the esophagus. The stomach acids may irritate the lining of the esophagus, causing a burning sensation known as heartburn. Heartburn may worsen during the second and third trimesters of pregnancy as the enlarging uterus pushes the stomach upward toward the esophagus.

How the immune response is altered during pregnancy

In response to foreign substances that enter the body, the immune system produces cells called T lymphocytes. These T lymphocytes would be expected to destroy "foreign" cells from the fetus that have entered the woman's bloodstream. However, the woman's immune system tolerates these fetal cells, possibly because she produces blocking antibodies during pregnancy. The blocking antibodies attach to the T lymphocytes and prevent them from attaching to and destroying the fetal cells.

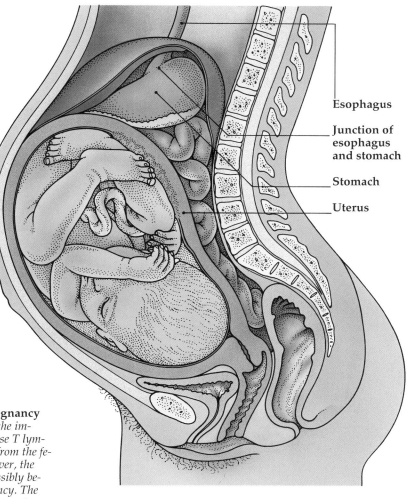

Esophagus

Junction of esophagus and stomach

Stomach

Uterus

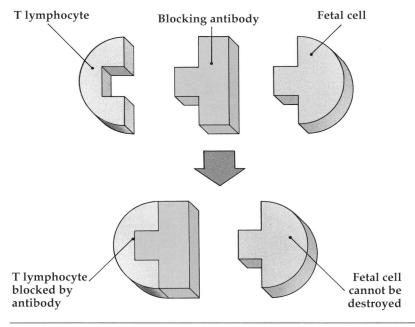

T lymphocyte

Blocking antibody

Fetal cell

T lymphocyte blocked by antibody

Fetal cell cannot be destroyed

IMMUNE SYSTEM

Your immune system usually attacks and destroys foreign substances, such as disease organisms, that enter your body. The responses of a pregnant woman's immune system to foreign substances are diminished, which may make her more susceptible to infections such as colds and the flu.

Cells of the fetus, which enter the woman's bloodstream during pregnancy, are also interpreted as foreign substances by the woman's immune system because they carry some proteins determined by the father's genes. But the woman's body tolerates the "foreign" cells of the fetus, perhaps because of an alteration in the effect of her immune system's response (see left).

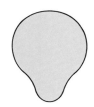 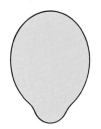

Uterus before pregnancy　　**Uterus at 8 weeks**　　**Uterus at 10 weeks**

The increasing size of the uterus
Beginning about week 12, when your doctor can feel the top of the uterus through your abdomen, he or she can use measurements of the height of your uterus above your pubic bone to monitor your pregnancy. Shown below are average heights of the uterus from 8 to 40 weeks of pregnancy. The height at 40 weeks decreases because the fetus drops downward in the pelvis in preparation for birth.

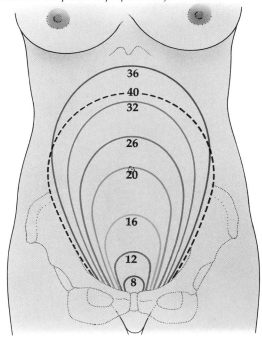

The changing shape of the uterus
In the first few weeks after conception, the uterus grows wider and changes from pear-shaped to almost round.

The female pelvis
The hipbones meet in front at a joint called the pubic symphysis. A woman's pubic symphysis is less rigid than a man's and her pelvis is shallower and wider. These differences facilitate childbirth. During pregnancy, the hormone relaxin, produced by the placenta, causes the connective tissues, ligaments, and joints (especially those in the pelvis) to become more flexible in preparation for childbirth. This flexibility may cause discomfort in the pelvic area, especially when walking (see ABDOMINAL PAIN on page 40).

THE UTERUS

During pregnancy, the blood supply to the uterus increases and the lining of the uterus (called the endometrium) softens and becomes thicker. Muscles in the wall of the uterus become stronger and more elastic; the muscle fibers increase in size by as much as 50 times. The uterus increases in weight from about 2 ounces before pregnancy to about 2 pounds just before delivery.

Throughout your pregnancy (and especially in the last few weeks), the muscles in the walls of the uterus contract gently at irregular intervals. These contractions (called Braxton Hicks contractions) are usually not painful and help circulate blood through the uterus.

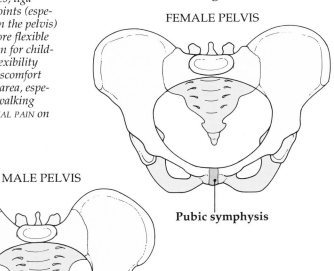

FEMALE PELVIS

MALE PELVIS

Pubic symphysis

OTHER BODY CHANGES

The increased level of progesterone during pregnancy causes your blood vessels to widen, bringing a greater supply of blood to body tissues. As a result of this increased blood supply, the tissues of your vagina, vulva (the external genital organs), and cervix (the neck of the uterus) may swell. Widening of the blood vessels in the legs and labia (the skin folds at the opening of the vagina) can lead to varicose (enlarged) veins (see page 45). Varicose veins usually shrink or disappear after the baby is born.

Glands in the cervix increase their secretion of mucus, resulting in a white discharge from the vagina. If the discharge changes in appearance or has an unpleasant odor, or if you experience itching or burning, consult your doctor (see URINARY TRACT INFECTIONS on page 45).

YOUR CHANGING SHAPE

When you are pregnant, your body shape is as distinctively yours as it was before you became pregnant – no two women's bodies change in exactly the same way.

First and second months
Your shape will not change a great deal and you may not notice a weight gain during the first 2 months. Your abdomen may appear to be slightly enlarged – not by growth of the uterus but because your intestines may be distended as a result of hormone changes. Your breasts may start to tingle and may be tender.

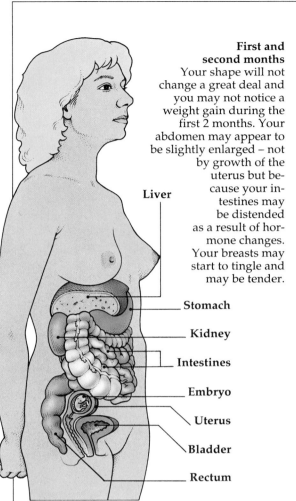

Liver

Stomach

Kidney

Intestines

Embryo

Uterus

Bladder

Rectum

Third and fourth months
Your abdomen begins to enlarge to accommodate the growing fetus and you usually gain about 3 or 4 pounds each month. Your breasts will continue to become fuller throughout your pregnancy, but the tenderness usually subsides. Colostrum (a fluid produced before breast milk) may be expressed from the nipples. The areolas (the pigmented areas around the nipples) and nipples darken, and veins start to become visible.

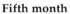
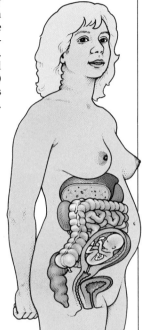

Fifth month
You may gain 3 to 4 pounds. You may notice that you begin to breathe more deeply and your heart rate increases. You may have swelling of your ankles and feet, and varicose (enlarged) veins may develop (see page 45). The areolas continue to darken and become wider.

Sixth and seventh months
During this period you gain weight rapidly. The skin over your abdomen becomes stretched and thin (see STRETCH MARKS on page 44). The uterus now extends above the level of your navel, displacing your abdominal organs. The pubic symphysis (the joint where the hipbones meet in the front of the pelvis) has widened.

Eighth month
You may gain 3 to 5 pounds. The uterus rises up under your diaphragm as the fetus turns head down. Your navel may flatten and then protrude.

Ninth month
With your first baby, the fetus's head settles ("drops") down farther into your pelvis in preparation for birth (this is called engagement – see page 90). If you have had a baby before, the head may not move down until you go into labor. You may feel more comfortable after the fetus has dropped, although you may notice a more frequent urge to urinate because of the increased pressure of the fetus's head on your bladder.

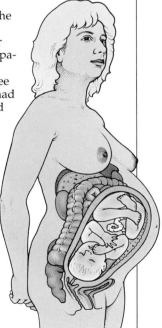

COMMON DISCOMFORTS DURING PREGNANCY

Even during a completely normal, healthy pregnancy, most women experience a variety of discomforts. These discomforts are usually temporary and do not indicate that you have a serious problem. If you are concerned about symptoms you are experiencing or if they become severe, talk to your doctor.

KEY

① 1st trimester
② 2nd trimester
③ 3rd trimester

ABDOMINAL PAIN

② ③

Symptoms
Sharp, shooting pains or cramps in your abdomen after sitting or lying in one position for a while, or a dull, aching pain in the lower part of the abdomen around the pelvic joints. Pain around your pelvic joints may worsen after walking or exercising.

Causes
Abdominal pain occurs when the ligaments that support your growing uterus stretch or pelvic joints loosen as a result of hormone changes.

Treatment or prevention
◆ Changing positions frequently when sitting or lying down may help relieve pain.
◆ Rest as often as possible and avoid any strenuous exercise.
◆ Consult your doctor if abdominal pain is severe, persistent, or accompanied by vaginal bleeding.

BACKACHE

① ② ③

Symptoms
Aching in the lower part of your back or the top of your buttocks.

Causes
The extra weight of the fetus in your abdomen causes you to lean back, putting a strain on the muscles and ligaments of your spine.

Treatment or prevention
◆ Do not gain more weight than recommended by your doctor.
◆ Exercise to strengthen the muscles in your back and abdomen.
◆ Sleep on a firm mattress.
◆ Wear low-heeled shoes.
◆ Do not lift heavy objects.

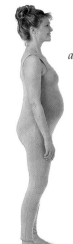

Good posture
Learn how to sit comfortably, without putting stress on your back muscles, and try to stand up straight to prevent your pelvis from tilting forward and the small of your back from curving inward.

BLEEDING GUMS

① ② ③

Symptoms
Bleeding gums when brushing your teeth or after eating.

Causes
Your gums become more sensitive and may swell as a result of the increased levels of some hormones.

Treatment or prevention
◆ See your dentist as early as possible in your pregnancy for a checkup. Your dentist will evaluate the need to perform or postpone any necessary dental work.

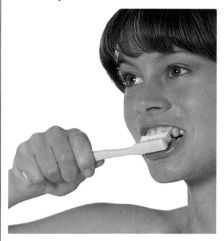

Keep your teeth clean
Be sure you brush and floss your teeth twice a day to prevent tooth decay and possible infection of your gums.

BREATHLESSNESS

③

Symptoms
Shortness of breath when you exert yourself or, in extreme cases, when you talk. Breathing may become more difficult when you lie down.

Causes
During the last few months of your pregnancy, the enlargement of the uterus puts pressure on your diaphragm, crowding your lungs. Your breathing may become easier during the last month of your pregnancy, when the fetus settles down farther in your pelvis.

Treatment or prevention
◆ Move slowly and avoid over-exerting yourself.
◆ Make a habit of sitting up straight.
◆ Use an extra pillow or two when you go to bed so that you sleep in a semireclining position.
◆ Consult your doctor if the shortness of breath suddenly becomes worse or is accompanied by any pain in your chest.

CARPAL TUNNEL SYNDROME

Symptoms
A pins-and-needles or burning sensation in your palm next to your thumb and first two fingers.

Causes
The extra amount of fluid in your body during pregnancy puts pressure on the median nerve as this nerve passes through a tunnel formed by the wrist bones (called the carpal tunnel). The problem should go away after the delivery.

Treatment or prevention
◆ To help relieve pain, elevate the affected hand or place the hand in cold water.
◆ Consult your doctor, who may recommend that you wear a splint on your wrist.

CONSTIPATION

Symptoms
Infrequent or difficult passage of hard, dry stools.

Causes
The hormone progesterone relaxes the muscles of the intestines, which slows the contractions that move stools through your bowels. When movement is slow, more water is absorbed, causing the stools to become hard and dry.

Treatment or prevention
◆ Exercise regularly.
◆ If you are taking iron tablets, take them after eating. They will be absorbed more easily and be less likely to aggravate constipation.
◆ Do not use laxatives or enemas.
◆ Drink six to eight glasses of liquids every day.
◆ Consult your doctor if the constipation persists.

Eat fiber-rich foods
Eat fiber-rich foods, such as fruit, nuts, vegetables, and whole-grain products.

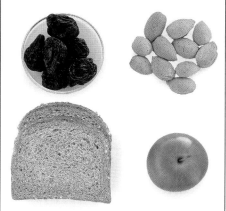

DIZZINESS OR FAINTING

Symptoms
Dizziness or feeling light-headed, especially when getting up from sitting or lying down.

Causes
During pregnancy, your blood pressure is lower. As a result, the flow of blood to your brain is reduced. You may feel dizzy or light-headed when you stand up because blood is suddenly, but temporarily, shifted away from your brain.

Treatment or prevention
◆ Avoid standing for long periods.
◆ Get up slowly after a warm bath or after sitting or lying down.
◆ Keep yourself as cool as possible during hot weather.
◆ Avoid hot, stuffy, crowded areas.

Feeling faint
Lie down with your feet elevated, or sit down and put your head between your knees. Lowering your head increases blood flow to your brain.

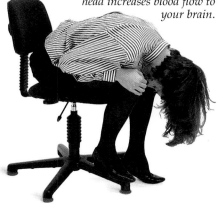

EYE PROBLEMS

Symptoms
Your vision may seem to worsen. If you wear contact lenses, they may become uncomfortable.

Causes
Retention of fluid may change the shape of your eyeball.

Treatment or prevention
◆ If you wear contact lenses, your doctor may recommend you stop wearing them during pregnancy.

Changes in vision
See your ophthalmologist if you think that your vision has changed.

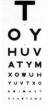
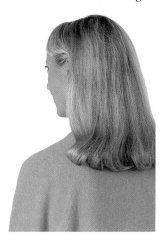

FLUID RETENTION

Symptoms
Your hands may swell and rings may no longer fit. Your ankles may swell and your shoes may feel tight.

Causes
The amount of fluid retained by the body increases during pregnancy.

Treatment or prevention
◆ Avoid standing for long periods.
◆ Rest with your legs elevated, especially toward the end of the day.
◆ Raise the bottom of your bed a few inches (do not do this if you are having heartburn).
◆ Avoid salty foods.
◆ Consult your doctor if the swelling becomes severe or you also have headaches or blurred vision.

FOOD CRAVINGS

Symptoms
You may experience strong cravings for some foods.

Causes
The cause of food cravings among pregnant women is not known, but may be related to the high level of progesterone in the body.

Treatment or prevention
◆ If you crave healthy foods, indulge yourself. If you crave foods that aren't good for you, consider a substitute or eat in moderation.
◆ Consult your doctor if you crave nonfood items such as paper or clay.

FREQUENT URINATION

Symptoms
You urinate more frequently than usual or often feel a strong urge to urinate but you pass only small amounts of urine.

Causes
Frequent urination may be caused by hormone activity, a higher fluid intake because of increased thirst, and the pressure of the enlarging uterus on the bladder.

Treatment or prevention
◆ Cut down on your intake of fluids shortly before you go to bed.
◆ Rocking backward and forward when urinating may help to empty your bladder more efficiently.
◆ Consult your doctor if you have pain when you urinate or your urine contains blood (see URINARY TRACT INFECTIONS on page 45).

GAS

Symptoms
Cramps in the abdomen, rumbling in the stomach, and bloating.

Causes
During pregnancy, sluggish bowel muscles may make it difficult to pass gas. Distention or spasm of the intestines may cause pain.

Treatment or prevention
◆ Chew your food well and eat slowly. Eating too fast causes you to swallow more air.
◆ Eat fiber-rich foods to avoid becoming constipated.
◆ Avoid fried and spicy food.
◆ Consult your doctor if the abdominal pain and bloating persist.

HEARTBURN

Symptoms
A burning pain in your chest behind the breastbone. The pain may worsen when you are lying down or just after you have eaten.

Causes
The muscle at the entrance to your stomach relaxes during pregnancy, allowing food that has mixed with stomach acid to be pushed upward into the esophagus.

Treatment or prevention
◆ Do not lie down for at least 2 hours after eating.
◆ Have a glass of milk just before going to bed.
◆ Sleep with the head of your bed elevated a few inches.
◆ Consult your doctor if the heartburn is severe or persists.

Watch your diet
Avoid overeating and don't eat spicy or fried foods, particularly late at night.

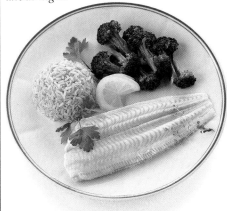

HEMORRHOIDS

Symptoms
Itching, soreness, and pain around the anus, and possibly blood when you have a bowel movement.

Causes
In the late stages of pregnancy, pressure from the uterus may cause hemorrhoids, which are swollen veins around your anus.

Treatment or prevention
◆ Eat high-fiber foods and drink plenty of liquids to avoid becoming constipated.

◆ Do not strain when having a bowel movement.

◆ Avoid standing or sitting for long periods of time.

◆ Keep the skin around your anus clean and dry.

◆ Warm baths twice a day may help relieve the discomfort.

◆ Consult your doctor if the discomfort persists or the hemorrhoids bleed. He or she may prescribe a hemorrhoid medication.

ITCHY SKIN

Symptoms
The skin over your abdomen itches.

Causes
The skin over your abdomen stretches as the uterus enlarges. As a result, the skin becomes taut and dry, leading to itching.

Treatment or prevention
◆ Apply a moisturizer or calamine lotion to help relieve the itching (try not to scratch).

◆ Consult your doctor if the itching affects your whole body.

LEAKAGE OF URINE

Symptoms
Leakage of urine when you cough, laugh, sneeze, or exert yourself.

Causes
The pressure of the enlarging uterus on your bladder and relaxation of the muscles in your pelvis may cause leakage of urine.

Treatment or prevention
◆ Urinate frequently.

◆ Practice pelvic floor exercises several times each day to help strengthen the pelvic muscles (see page 66).

◆ Consult your doctor if the problem persists after delivery.

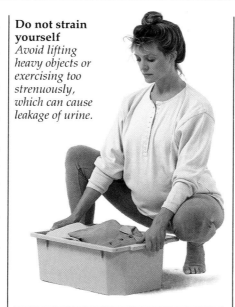

Do not strain yourself
Avoid lifting heavy objects or exercising too strenuously, which can cause leakage of urine.

LEG CRAMPS

Symptoms
Sharp pains in the muscles in your calves or thighs, often followed by a dull ache that lasts several hours.

Causes
Muscle cramps may be caused by the increased pressure of the uterus on blood vessels that carry blood to your legs or by a calcium deficiency.

Treatment or prevention
◆ Firmly massage or apply heat to the affected area to help relieve pain.

◆ Gently work a painful calf muscle by straightening your leg and flexing your ankle and toes upward.

◆ Consult your doctor if the muscle cramps persist.

MORNING SICKNESS

Symptoms
You may feel nauseated and vomit.

Causes
The increased levels of hormones during pregnancy may cause morning sickness (see pages 26 and 27).

Treatment or prevention
◆ Eat and drink something before you get out of bed in the morning.

◆ Eat small, frequent meals.

◆ Do not get overtired; fatigue may make nausea worse.

◆ Consult your doctor if vomiting becomes severe.

NASAL STUFFINESS AND NOSEBLEEDS

Symptoms
A stuffy nose, sometimes accompanied by nosebleeds.

Causes
The increased level of the hormone estrogen and the increased blood supply during pregnancy cause the mucous membranes in your nose to swell, resulting in stuffiness. The increased blood supply also causes blood vessels in the lining of the nose to swell. Strenuous or frequent blowing of your nose may cause small blood vessels to burst.

Treatment or prevention
◆ Blow your nose gently.

◆ Do not use a nasal spray unless it is prescribed by your doctor.

◆ A vaporizer or humidifier may help keep the nasal membranes moist, making the membranes less likely to split and bleed.

Stopping a nosebleed
Sit down, lower your chin slightly toward your chest, and pinch your nostrils firmly together for about 15 minutes.

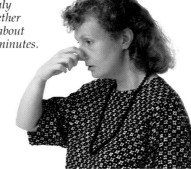

PIGMENTATION CHANGES

Symptoms

Darkening of your nipples and areolas (the dark areas around your nipples) and a dark line down the middle of your abdomen are normal. The color of freckles or birthmarks may deepen.

Causes

Changes in hormone levels result in increased production of pigment-producing cells. Sunlight may intensify changes in pigmentation.

Treatment or prevention

◆ Do not attempt to bleach your skin. Most of the unusual pigmentation will fade soon after delivery.

Stay out of the sun
Sit in the shade, cover up, and apply a sunscreen on sunny days. Do not use a sunlamp or tanning bed.

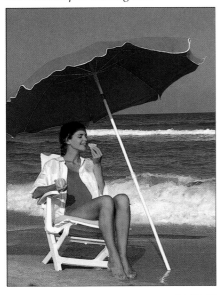

RASHES

Symptoms

A red, scaly rash in skin folds (such as under the breasts or in the groin).

Causes

Rashes in skin folds are caused by the skin surfaces rubbing together.

Treatment or prevention

◆ Avoid gaining excessive weight.
◆ Keep affected areas clean and dry.
◆ Consult your doctor if the rash persists or shows signs of infection.

RIB PAIN

Symptoms

Soreness and tenderness in the area of the ribs under your breasts.

Causes

As the uterus enlarges and expands upward into your chest, it causes pressure against your ribs. The pain usually disappears when the fetus settles down lower in the pelvis.

Treatment or prevention

◆ Avoid putting pressure on your ribs; when resting or sleeping, lie in a semireclining position.

SCIATICA

Symptoms

Pains that shoot from the lower part of your back and buttocks down the backs of your legs. The shooting pains are often accompanied by a pins-and-needles sensation.

Causes

The sciatic nerves in your pelvis are being compressed by the uterus.

Treatment or prevention

◆ Rest as much as possible and avoid strenuous exercise.
◆ Adjust your body position (for example, lie on your side rather than on your back) to try to decrease the pressure on the pelvic nerves.
◆ Consult your doctor if the back and leg pains are severe.

STRETCH MARKS

Symptoms

Red lines (stretch marks) on the skin of your abdomen, breasts, or thighs. Stretch marks do not disappear completely, but will gradually fade.

Causes

These marks are caused by the stretching of your skin.

Treatment or prevention

◆ Avoid gaining excessive weight; this can sometimes help avoid stretch marks.

SWEATING

Symptoms

Excessive perspiration after little or no exertion. You may wake up at night feeling hot and sweaty.

Causes

Hormone changes cause the blood vessels just below the skin surface to widen. The blood flow to the skin increases, producing heat. Sweating is the body's way of cooling itself.

Treatment or prevention

◆ Wear loose-fitting cotton clothes.
◆ Drink plenty of liquids.
◆ Sleep in a cool room.

Shower or bathe frequently
Frequent baths or showers help keep you feeling fresh and cool.

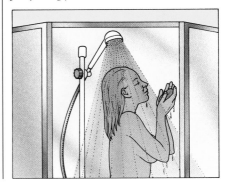

TASTE CHANGES

Symptoms
You may have a metallic taste in your mouth, making foods taste unpleasant or different than usual.

Causes
The causes of taste changes are unknown, but may be related to the increased hormone activity.

Treatment or prevention
◆ Eat whatever nutritious foods taste good to you.

TIREDNESS

Symptoms
You may find that you feel so tired that you need a nap during the day.

Causes
Tiredness is a normal part of pregnancy, caused by the extra demands on your body. Sometimes excessive fatigue is the result of worry, lack of sleep, or poor nutrition.

Treatment or prevention
◆ Get plenty of sleep and rest when you feel tired.
◆ Exercise regularly.
◆ Eat a well-balanced diet.

URINARY TRACT INFECTIONS

Symptoms
An urge to urinate often (even when you have just finished urinating); pain or burning when you urinate. Your urine may be cloudy, smelly, or spotted with blood.

Causes
Urinary tract infections are common during pregnancy. Relaxation of the muscles in the urinary tract and retention of fluids make it easier for bacteria to cause infections.

Treatment or prevention
◆ Consult your doctor immediately. He or she will test your urine and prescribe antibiotics.

Drink cranberry juice
If you have a urinary tract infection, in addition to prescribing antibiotics, your doctor may recommend you drink large quantities of liquids, particularly cranberry juice, because it provides acidity to help fight the infection.

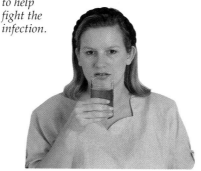

VAGINAL DISCHARGE

Symptoms
A thin, white discharge from the vagina during pregnancy is normal (see OTHER BODY CHANGES on page 38). A discharge that appears yellowish or greenish, has an unpleasant odor, becomes thick and cheesy, or is accompanied by itching or burning indicates an infection.

Causes
During pregnancy, the higher levels of hormones cause an increased production of mucus and changes within the vagina that allow some organisms to multiply rapidly.

Treatment or prevention
◆ Keep your genital area clean and as dry as possible.
◆ Wear loose-fitting cotton – not nylon – underpants.
◆ Do not wear panty hose or pants that are tight.

◆ Avoid using scented or deodorant soaps, vaginal deodorants, or douches, which may irritate the tissues in your vaginal area.
◆ Consult your doctor if you think you might have a vaginal infection. If necessary, he or she will prescribe medication – usually a vaginal cream or suppositories.

VARICOSE VEINS

Symptoms
Aching pain in your legs, often with itchy or irritated skin. The leg veins may swell and appear dark purple. You may also have a heavy feeling in your labia (the skin folds at the opening to the vagina).

Causes
The increased pressure of the uterus on the veins in your pelvis, legs, and labia causes blood to accumulate in these veins. This accumulated blood stretches the veins and breaks down the valves that prevent backflow. As a result, varicose veins sometimes develop. If your family has a history of varicose veins, you are more likely to develop them.

Treatment or prevention
◆ Avoid excessive weight gain.
◆ Avoid standing for long periods.
◆ Wear support stockings.
◆ Take a walk every day.

Elevate your legs
When sitting or lying down, elevate your legs.

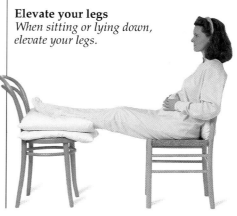

CHAPTER THREE

PRENATAL CARE

ONE OF THE FIRST and most important decisions you will make as you prepare for your new baby is the choice of a health care professional for prenatal care and delivery. Choose a doctor or nurse-midwife you like and trust – someone who shares your views on pregnancy and childbirth and also understands your concerns. It is very important that you make this decision as early as possible during your pregnancy. Prenatal care that is started early and continues throughout your pregnancy (usually once a month during the first 6 months and then more frequently during the last 3 months) will help ensure that you have a healthy pregnancy and that your baby will have the best possible start in life. In this chapter, we explain each of the tests that you will have during your prenatal visits. We also discuss several optional tests that your doctor may rec-

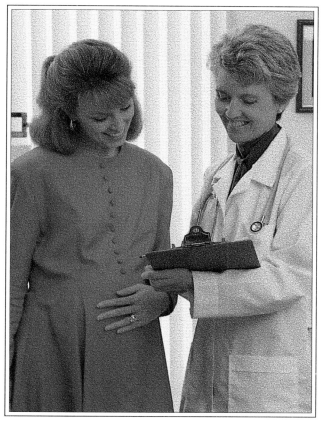

ommend in some special circumstances. A well-balanced diet, regular exercise, and a healthy life-style are always important, but especially during pregnancy. Eating well and not drinking alcohol or smoking are essential to the growth and well-being of the fetus. Staying physically fit helps make your pregnancy more comfortable and helps you cope with the physical demands of labor and delivery. To help prepare for childbirth and parenthood, you and your partner may want to attend childbirth education classes. These classes teach you what to expect during your pregnancy, labor, and delivery, as well as how to care for your newborn baby. Many childbirth education classes include instruction on exercises and breathing and relaxation techniques for you to use during labor and delivery.

Most pregnancies progress without complications. Early and regular prenatal care allows your doctor or nurse-midwife to detect possible warning signs of a problem, and most problems can be treated before they become serious. Women who have certain medical conditions (diabetes and asthma, for example) require particularly close monitoring during their pregnancies because they are at an increased risk of complications. In the final section of this chapter, we discuss two serious complications of pregnancy – miscarriage and ectopic pregnancy (a pregnancy that occurs outside the uterus, usually in a fallopian tube). Some miscarriages can be prevented and the pregnancy can continue. An ectopic pregnancy must be terminated immediately by surgery. Both of these complications tend to occur in the first few months of pregnancy, so early prenatal care is essential to ensure prompt diagnosis and proper treatment.

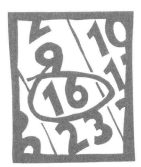

PLANNING FOR CHILDBIRTH

O NLY 50 YEARS AGO, a pregnant woman had few choices in the care she received at childbirth. Today, the role of expectant parents has changed significantly – from that of spectators to active decision-makers. You and your partner can make many decisions about how your pregnancy, labor, and delivery will be managed.

Your choices and decisions
Before you and your partner make any decisions about the birth of your baby, you may want to make a list of your personal requirements and preferences about labor and delivery. You may also want to list any questions you would like to discuss with your doctor.

When planning for childbirth, your most important choices will include selecting the person who will provide your health care, what method of childbirth you want (see CHILDBIRTH EDUCATION CLASSES on page 67), and where you want to deliver your baby. Each of these decisions may influence the others. For example, the method of childbirth you want may influence your choice of health care professional and where you have your baby. You should make these decisions as early as possible in your pregnancy – after carefully considering all of your requirements and options – to ensure a healthy pregnancy and comfortable labor and delivery.

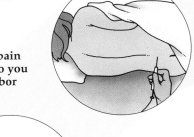

What types of pain relief, if any, do you want during labor and delivery?

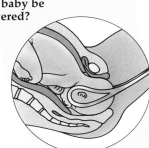

Where will your baby be delivered?

What type of care is right for you?
In the process of making your decisions about childbirth, many questions and concerns arise. Your doctor, partner, relatives and friends can provide guidance and support.

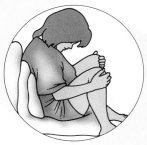

How much medical intervention do you want? Under what circumstances would a cesarean, a forceps delivery, or an episiotomy be acceptable?

What position do you want to use to deliver your baby?

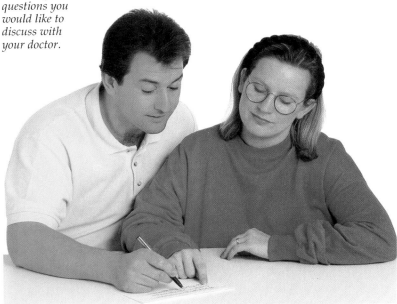

CHOOSING A HEALTH CARE PROFESSIONAL

Most babies in the US are delivered by obstetricians or by family practitioners. Some women feel more comfortable with a certified nurse-midwife. When choosing your health care professional, you should consider his or her reputation with other patients and doctors, fees, office hours, and the location of the hospital where he or she practices. When you have found a prospective doctor or nurse-midwife, arrange a get-acquainted visit to ask about his or her approach to childbirth – for example, what method of childbirth preparation he or she prefers and why; how he or she feels about pain medication during labor; whether he or she routinely performs episiotomies (cutting of the tissue between the vaginal opening and the anus); and in what percentage of births he or she induces labor, uses forceps for delivery, or performs a cesarean section. You should discuss your ideas and preferences about how you want your pregnancy and delivery to be managed. If the doctor or nurse-midwife is not sympathetic to your plans and wishes, or you do not feel at ease with him or her, keep looking.

Who will be your health care professional? Do you prefer a doctor or a nurse-midwife?

Will other family members, including the baby's brothers and sisters, be able to visit at the hospital?

Will your partner be present during labor and delivery?

Will it be possible to hold and/or breast-feed your baby immediately after delivery?

What method of preparation for childbirth do you want?

Obstetricians and family practitioners

An obstetrician is a doctor who has received specialized training in the care of women during pregnancy, labor, and childbirth. Some obstetricians (called perinatologists) specialize in high-risk pregnancies – for example, women with conditions such as diabetes or with a family history of a genetic (inherited) disorder. A family practitioner is a doctor who has received additional training in primary medicine, including obstetrics. If complications occur during your pregnancy, a family practitioner may refer you to an obstetrician.

A certified nurse-midwife

A pregnant woman who is at low risk for complications may select a certified nurse-midwife as her health care professional. A certified nurse-midwife is a registered nurse who has undergone obstetric training limited to managing a normal, uncomplicated pregnancy and labor. In many states, a certified nurse-midwife must practice in association with a doctor (that is, a doctor serves as a backup if problems arise).

KEY

A Heart rate and blood pressure monitor

B Anesthetic outlet

C Oxygen outlet

D Electronic fetal monitor

E Instrument table

F Baby crib and warmer

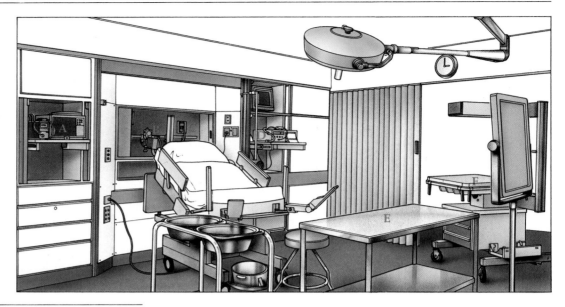

WHERE TO HAVE YOUR BABY

In the US, the majority of deliveries take place in a hospital (in a delivery room or birthing room) or in a birthing center. Some women choose to give birth at home. When choosing where you want to deliver your baby, carefully assess the risks and benefits of each type of birth setting. It is important that you consider the level of medical care that each is equipped to provide so that you ensure the safest possible labor and delivery for both you and your baby. Talk to your health care professional to help determine what type of birth setting would be most appropriate for you.

The hospital

Hospital policies on labor and delivery vary – from traditional to very flexible. Be sure to make an appointment with the hospital of your choice for a tour of the maternity unit. Ask lots of questions. For example, you may want to know whether the hospital offers childbirth education classes; what methods of childbirth the staff is familiar with; what kind of monitoring techniques will be available during your labor; whether your partner can be present during the birth; and what the hospital-acquired infection rate is.

The birthing center

A birthing center provides a relaxed, homelike, family-oriented environment for women at low risk of having complications during labor and delivery. A birthing center may be in a hospital or may be a separate facility. Regulations for free-standing birthing centers vary by state; you should check to see if a center has been licensed by the state or accredited by a national association. Care is provided mainly by certified nurse-midwives who work in consultation with obstetricians. If complications arise during the birth, the doctor-on-call will take over or you may be transferred to a hospital.

Your home

Some women prefer home birth as a more natural alternative to the traditional hospital setting. If you are considering a home birth, discuss the risks, benefits, and alternatives with the health care professional who will deliver your baby.

The hospital delivery room
The hospital delivery room is specifically equipped for delivery. High-technology medical equipment is available, if needed, in case complications arise.

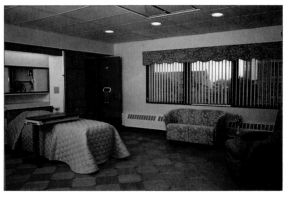

The birthing room
A hospital birthing room is a private room in which a woman experiences labor, delivery, and recovery. It helps provide a natural, homelike setting and a relaxed atmosphere.

YOUR CHOICES FOR PAIN RELIEF

Medications given for the relief of pain during labor and delivery have different risks and benefits for the woman and the baby. You should discuss the types of pain relief you prefer with your health care professional. For more information, see HOW PAIN MEDICATIONS ARE GIVEN DURING LABOR AND DELIVERY on page 96).

Regional anesthetics

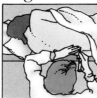

An epidural block is a type of regional anesthesia commonly used to relieve pain during labor and delivery. An anesthetic is injected through your back into the space between the vertebrae and the membranes covering your spinal cord (called the epidural space). A small tube (called a catheter) is inserted into the injection site and comfortably remains there throughout labor and delivery, allowing for additional medication to be given if it is needed. The anesthetic affects nerves that lead to the chest and the lower half of the body, relieving labor pains. An epidural anesthetic does not reach your brain (so you will not feel drowsy) or the baby's bloodstream.

Local anesthetics

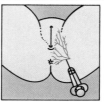

A pudendal block is an anesthetic used to relieve pain in the vagina and perineum (the tissues between the vaginal opening and anus) during delivery. The anesthetic is injected into the area of the pudendal nerve on each side of the lower part of the pelvis, either through the walls of the vagina or through the perineum. For an episiotomy (see page 109), a local anesthetic may be injected just under the skin where the incision is to be made.

Analgesics

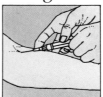

Analgesics are painkillers that are given by injection or intravenous infusion. Analgesics given in either of these ways reach all parts of the body, including the brain, relieving labor pain and helping the woman relax. Meperidine, a narcotic drug, is an analgesic commonly given for pain relief during childbirth, although morphine or other narcotics are sometimes used.

Prepared childbirth

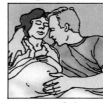

Some women prefer to have their babies with little or no anesthesia or pain-killing drugs, no episiotomy, and no use of forceps – known as prepared (or natural) childbirth. Childbirth education classes (see page 67) help prepare expectant parents by providing information about pregnancy, labor, and delivery and teaching various techniques (most common is the Lamaze method) to help a woman cope with the demands of labor and delivery. The information given in the classes helps to reduce fear; the breathing and relaxation techniques help to relieve tension. A less fearful, less tense woman is usually better prepared to cope with pain.

Getting prepared
Some hospitals and most birthing centers offer childbirth education classes (see page 67). You and your partner learn about the birth process and topics such as bathing the baby, breast-feeding, and how to put on a diaper. You also learn breathing and relaxation techniques to help you during your labor and delivery.

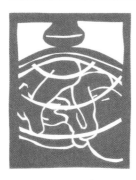

TESTS AND EXAMINATIONS

RENATAL CARE is the health care you receive before your baby is born. During your prenatal visits, your doctor will perform tests and examinations to assess both your well-being and that of the developing fetus. Early and regularly scheduled prenatal care is essential to help prevent problems or to detect them as soon as possible so that they can be treated most effectively.

As soon as you suspect that you might be pregnant, you should make an appointment to see your doctor. If the pregnancy is confirmed, your doctor will schedule you for regular checkups throughout your pregnancy.

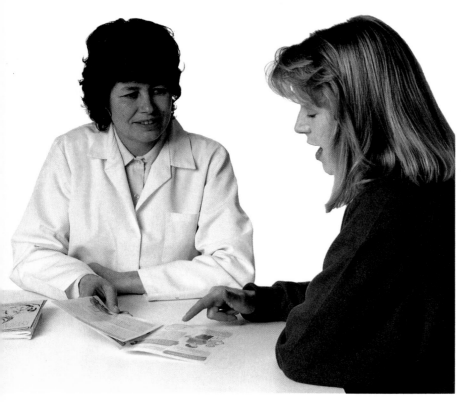

An opportunity for discussion
At your first prenatal visit, your doctor will explain the various tests and examinations that will be performed. Be sure to ask questions about any tests you don't understand or about symptoms you may be experiencing. Remember there is no such thing as a foolish question.

YOUR FIRST PRENATAL VISIT

Your first prenatal visit is the most thorough. Your doctor will ask questions about your personal and family medical history, your diet and life-style, and the symptoms of pregnancy you are experiencing. The doctor will also perform a physical examination and order tests to check your current state of health.

Your gynecological history
To assess your pregnancy and determine the age of the fetus, your doctor will want to know the first day of your last menstrual period and the dates and results of pregnancy tests that you may have already had. Your doctor will also want to know certain details of your gynecological history that could influence your pregnancy. Such information will include the date of your last cervical (Pap) smear and what treatments you received if you have had abnormal Pap smears; whether you have a history of fibroids (noncancerous tumors of the uterus – see page 69), infections of the pelvic organs, or any abnormal vaginal discharge; and whether you have had previous pregnancies (including abortions and miscarriages), infertility tests and treatments, or surgery on your ovaries or uterus.

YOUR PRENATAL TESTS

The table below outlines the examinations and tests you may have during your pregnancy.

	AT YOUR FIRST VISIT	AT YOUR REGULAR VISITS
Physical examination 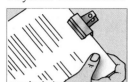	To assess heart and lungs; check blood pressure; examine abdomen and pelvis (an internal examination); perform a cervical (Pap) smear; measure weight and height.	To measure weight; check blood pressure; examine abdomen (to check growth of the fetus); check the fetus's heartbeat with an ultrasound device (from 10 to 12 weeks onward) or a stethoscope (from 20 to 24 weeks onward); check for signs of swelling of hands or ankles.
Urine tests 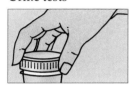	To measure glucose (sugar) levels (to check for possible diabetes); test for blood or protein (indicating kidney disease or infection); confirm the pregnancy.	To check the level of glucose and for the presence of blood or protein.
Blood tests 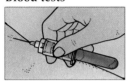	To measure levels of hemoglobin, the oxygen-carrying substance in red blood cells (to check for anemia); find out your blood group (see page 55); check for rubella (German measles) immunity; check for exposure to the hepatitis B virus or a sexually transmitted disease.	To measure hemoglobin levels; check for Rh (Rhesus) antibodies against the fetus's red blood cells (which may be produced if you are Rh negative and your partner and the fetus are Rh positive – see HOW THE Rh FACTOR CAN AFFECT PREGNANCY on page 79).

TESTS THAT ARE PERFORMED IF NECESSARY

Urine and blood tests
To check for abnormal levels of alpha-fetoprotein, which can indicate spina bifida (if too high) or Down's syndrome (if too low); check glucose levels to determine if you have gestational diabetes (diabetes during pregnancy) – see GLUCOSE SCREENING TEST on page 56; assess functioning of the placenta and the well-being of the fetus.

Amniocentesis
To measure alpha-fetoprotein (AFP) levels in the amniotic fluid if the blood AFP levels are abnormal (to detect the developmental abnormality spina bifida); to detect chromosome abnormalities such as Down's syndrome.

Ultrasound scanning
To determine the age of the fetus; detect more than one fetus; assess position, growth, and development of the fetus; locate the placenta; assess the amount of amniotic fluid; perform chorionic villus sampling, amniocentesis, or fetal blood sampling.

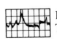

Fetal blood sampling
To check that the fetus is normal; to decide about a blood transfusion if the fetus is anemic as a result of Rh antibodies attacking its blood cells (see YOUR BLOOD GROUP on page 55 and HOW THE Rh FACTOR CAN AFFECT PREGNANCY on page 79).

Chorionic villus sampling
To analyze cells taken from the placenta (to detect chromosome abnormalities such as Down's syndrome or some inherited disorders such as cystic fibrosis).

Electronic fetal heart rate monitoring
To check the fetus's heartbeat.

Your medical history

You should tell your doctor about any medical problems you have had in the past and any current or long-term medical conditions (such as high blood pressure or diabetes). This information is important because some medical conditions can have an effect on your pregnancy and some can be adversely affected by the pregnancy. Pregnancy increases the work load on the heart, kidneys, and lungs. If these organs have been weakened by a previous or current condition, monitoring and treatment may be needed. You should also mention any operations you have had.

Tell your doctor if you have had a sexually transmitted disease (such as gonorrhea, herpes, or syphilis) or if you suspect you may be infected with the human immunodeficiency virus (HIV, the virus that causes AIDS). Sexually transmitted diseases and HIV may be transmitted to the fetus while it is in the uterus or during delivery.

Medications and drugs

Medications and drugs can adversely affect the fetus. Tell your doctor about any medications you take regularly, as well as any drugs (legal or illegal, including alcohol and marijuana) or medications that you have taken or used, even once, since you've been pregnant. Use of an illegal narcotic drug (such as heroin) can cause a baby to have severe breathing difficulties at birth. The baby may need to be treated or to be carefully withdrawn from the drug. Cocaine may cause poor fetal growth, birth defects, premature labor, severe bleeding from the placenta, or even death of the fetus.

Your family medical history

Your doctor will ask you whether anyone in your family or your partner's family has an inherited disorder such as sickle cell disease (a form of anemia) or hemophilia (a bleeding disorder).

PHYSICAL EXAMINATION

At your first prenatal visit, your doctor will perform a complete physical examination to assess your general health (see below). The doctor will do an internal (pelvic) examination (see page 29) to check your abdominal and pelvic organs and to assess the growth of your uterus and the size and shape of your pelvis. You will also have a cervical (Pap) smear if you have not had one in the past year.

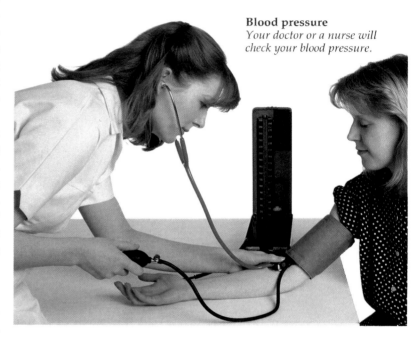

Blood pressure
Your doctor or a nurse will check your blood pressure.

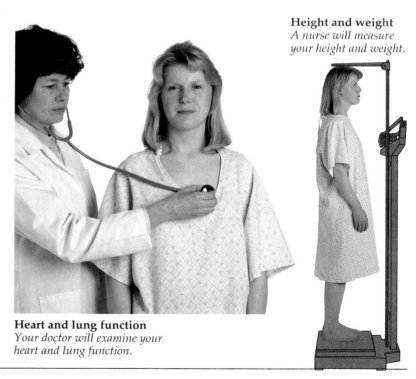

Height and weight
A nurse will measure your height and weight.

Heart and lung function
Your doctor will examine your heart and lung function.

Urine tests

When you make an appointment for your first prenatal visit, you will be asked to provide a sample of your urine. A nurse will perform a pregnancy test on this sample. The nurse will also test the sample for glucose (a sugar), albumin (a protein that is not normally found in urine), and blood. Glucose in your urine can be a sign of diabetes, which may require treatment to prevent possible problems during your pregnancy. Albumin or blood in your urine can indicate a urinary tract infection or kidney problems. If albumin or blood is present in your urine, your doctor will perform additional tests to diagnose the problem and start proper treatment.

BLOOD TESTS

At your first prenatal visit, your doctor will order a number of blood tests. In addition to the tests described below, your blood sample may be tested for a hormone called human chorionic gonadotropin to confirm your pregnancy.

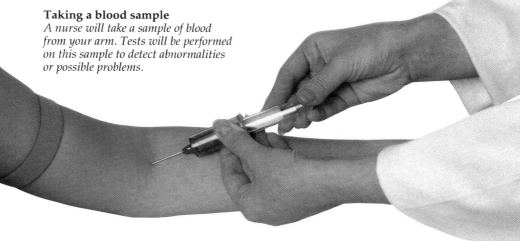

Taking a blood sample
A nurse will take a sample of blood from your arm. Tests will be performed on this sample to detect abnormalities or possible problems.

Your hemoglobin level
Hemoglobin is the substance in red blood cells that transports oxygen. During pregnancy, your hemoglobin level may fall slightly as a result of the increased volume of fluids in your body. If your hemoglobin level is too low, you may need treatment for anemia.

Your blood group
Your blood group (A, B, or O) will be determined in case a blood transfusion is needed. Your blood will also be checked for the Rh (Rhesus) factor, and a blood test called an antibody screen will be done to see if Rh antibodies (or other unusual antibodies) are present (see page 79).

Test for rubella immunity
If you become infected with the rubella (German measles) virus during pregnancy, the disease can cause serious problems (such as cataracts and deafness) in the fetus. If you have not had rubella or been vaccinated, you are susceptible. Because the vaccine should not be given during pregnancy, avoid contact with anyone who has the infection.

Test for the hepatitis B virus
Your blood will be tested for the hepatitis B virus. The virus can be present in your bloodstream without causing any symptoms. If the virus is present, it can be passed to your baby during delivery. To prevent hepatitis infections from developing in babies born to women infected with the virus, immunization is started right after birth.

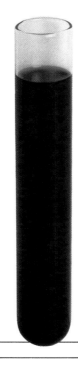

Tests for syphilis and HIV
Your blood will be tested for syphilis. If syphilis is not treated with antibiotics, the infection can have serious effects on the fetus. Your doctor may also advise you to be tested for HIV (the virus that causes AIDS).

Test for abnormal types of hemoglobin
If you are black, Asian, or of Mediterranean descent, your blood may be tested for abnormal types of hemoglobin, which are present in inherited disorders such as sickle cell disease or thalassemia (forms of anemia – see page 83). These conditions can worsen during pregnancy. The fetus may also be affected.

YOUR REGULAR VISITS

Throughout your pregnancy, your doctor will monitor your health and the health and growth of the fetus. You will usually be scheduled to see your doctor once a month for the first 28 weeks, every 2 weeks up to week 36, and then once a week until delivery.

At your regular visits, the nurse will check your weight and blood pressure; urine and blood tests may also be done (see YOUR PRENATAL TESTS on page 53). Your doctor will do an internal (pelvic) examination to check that your pregnancy is progressing normally.

OPTIONAL TESTS

A pregnant woman who is at risk of having a baby with an abnormality (see WHAT CAN GO WRONG? on page 57) may be advised to have additional tests to check that the fetus is normal. Ask your doctor to explain the risks and benefits of the tests before you decide to have them.

Alpha-fetoprotein testing

Alpha-fetoprotein (AFP) is a normal protein produced by the fetus. Some of the AFP passes into the woman's bloodstream by way of the placenta. A sample of the woman's blood may be tested to determine the AFP level. Results of this test are most accurate when it is done between weeks 16 and 18. Abnormally high levels of AFP may indicate that the fetus has a neural tube defect (a failure of the spine or brain to develop normally). Abnormally low AFP levels in the blood can be an indication that the fetus has Down's syndrome.

Amniocentesis

Amniocentesis is a procedure used to remove a sample of the amniotic fluid for analysis (see right). If recommended, amniocentesis is usually done between the 16th and 18th weeks of pregnancy.

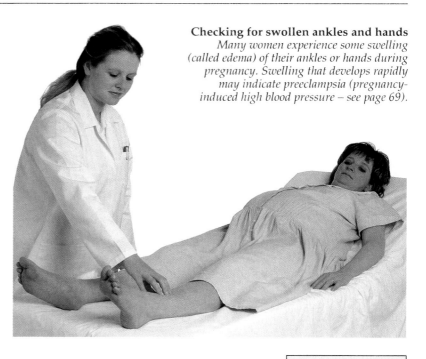

Checking for swollen ankles and hands
Many women experience some swelling (called edema) of their ankles or hands during pregnancy. Swelling that develops rapidly may indicate preeclampsia (pregnancy-induced high blood pressure – see page 69).

Amniocentesis is commonly done if a woman is over 35 years old or has an abnormal result from an AFP blood test. Fetal cells in the amniotic fluid can be analyzed to detect chromosome abnormalities or single-gene disorders (see page 57). Amniocentesis carries a very

Taking a sample of the amniotic fluid
Amniocentesis is done under the guidance of ultrasound (see page 58). An anesthetic is injected into the skin over the abdomen. A needle is inserted through the abdomen into the amniotic sac. A sample of the amniotic fluid is withdrawn into a syringe.

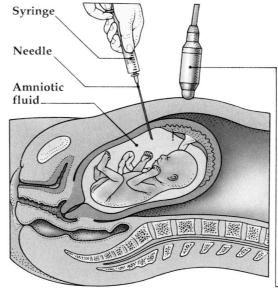

Syringe

Needle

Amniotic fluid

Ultrasound transducer

GLUCOSE SCREENING TEST

Many doctors perform a blood test called a glucose screening test at a prenatal visit to check for a temporary condition called gestational diabetes (diabetes during pregnancy). The test is usually done during weeks 24 to 28 – or earlier if there is a family history of diabetes. You will be asked to drink a solution that is high in glucose (a sugar). One hour later a blood sample will be taken to check the level of glucose. If the glucose level is too high, you may have gestational diabetes. Your doctor may order additional tests.

small risk (about 0.5 percent) of causing a miscarriage. Amniocentesis is considered a safer, more accurate procedure than chorionic villus sampling.

Chorionic villus sampling

Chorionic villus sampling (CVS) is the removal of tissue from the placenta for analysis (see right). This procedure can be performed as early as the sixth week. CVS may be done if the fetus is at high risk of having an abnormality or when detection of an abnormality must be made as early as possible if termination of the pregnancy is being considered. The risk of harming the fetus by CVS is higher than by amniocentesis, and CVS has a higher risk (about 2 percent) of miscarriage than amniocentesis.

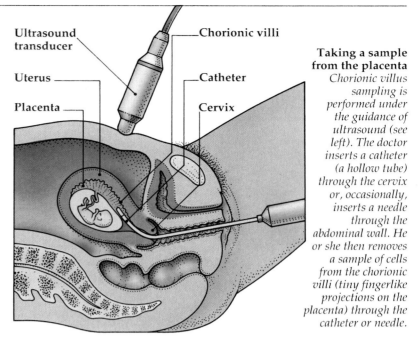

Taking a sample from the placenta
Chorionic villus sampling is performed under the guidance of ultrasound (see left). The doctor inserts a catheter (a hollow tube) through the cervix or, occasionally, inserts a needle through the abdominal wall. He or she then removes a sample of cells from the chorionic villi (tiny fingerlike projections on the placenta) through the catheter or needle.

WHAT CAN GO WRONG?

Some women may be at an increased risk of having a baby with a particular abnormality. These abnormalities can be classified as chromosome disorders, developmental disorders, or single-gene disorders.

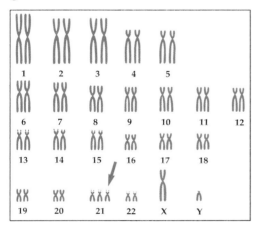

Chromosome disorders
A chromosome disorder is a disease that occurs as a result of a change in the number or structure of the chromosomes. The most common chromosome disorder is Down's syndrome, in which the cells contain an extra copy of chromosome number 21 (arrow). The risk of having a baby with Down's syndrome, as with most chromosome disorders, increases in women who become pregnant in their late 30s or 40s.

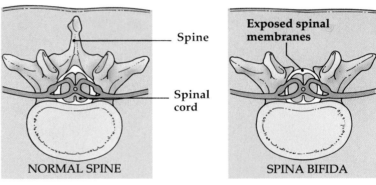

NORMAL SPINE   SPINA BIFIDA

Developmental disorders
A small percentage of fetuses fail to develop normally. Spina bifida (failure of the bones of the spine to close – shown above right in cross section) is one of the most common types of developmental abnormalities, occurring in one or two babies in every 1,000 live births. A woman who has had one affected child is 10 times more likely than the average to have another affected child.

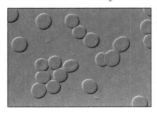
Normal red blood cells

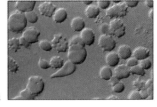
Thalassemia

Single-gene disorders
Single-gene disorders are caused by defects in a single pair of genes. These disorders may result from a child inheriting a single copy of an abnormal gene from one parent or two copies of an abnormal gene (one from each parent). Such a disorder can also occur if a parent's egg or sperm has a new mutation (a change in its genetic material). Examples of single-gene disorders are hemophilia (a bleeding disorder) and thalassemia (a form of anemia). Shown above are thalassemic (right) and normal (left) red blood cells.

ULTRASOUND SCANNING

Ultrasound scanning uses energy in the form of sound waves directed into a specific part of the body. The sound waves are reflected off internal organs (and, during pregnancy, off the fetus) and are converted into an image on a monitor. These sound waves are not harmful to the fetus or to the woman. Your doctor may recommend an ultrasound scan for one or more of the reasons described below and at right.

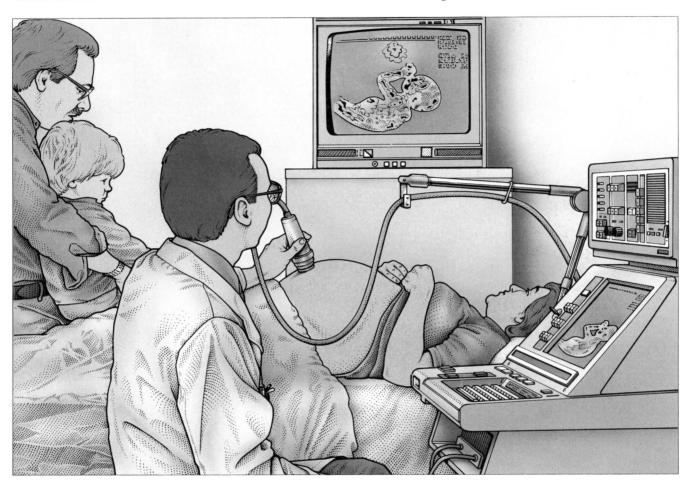

**To check the
size of the fetus**
An ultrasound scan may be done to check the size of the fetus, enabling the doctor to estimate its age. Your doctor may be unable to accurately determine the age of the fetus by other means if, for example, you are unsure of the date of your last menstrual period or if you stopped taking oral contraceptives just before you became pregnant.

**To detect the
fetus's heartbeat**
The fetus's heart is visible with ultrasound as early as 6 weeks after the last menstrual period. Beginning around the 10th to 12th week of pregnancy, Doppler ultrasound – a form of ultrasound that detects movement (including the flow of blood within blood vessels) – can be used to monitor the fetus's heartbeat.

**If you experience vaginal
bleeding or unusual pain
during pregnancy**
If you have any vaginal bleeding or unusual pain during pregnancy, an ultrasound scan may be done to confirm that the fetus is growing in the uterus and not in a fallopian tube (called an ectopic pregnancy) and to check the well-being of the fetus and the position of the placenta on the wall of the uterus.

**To identify
the fetus's position**
If the fetus's position is difficult to determine, ultrasound may be used. For most of your pregnancy, the fetus's head is toward the top of the uterus. Near the end of your pregnancy, the fetus usually turns so that its head is pointing downward in preparation for birth. Doctors are usually able to confirm fetal position by physical examination.

To guide amniocentesis, chorionic villus sampling, or fetal blood sampling

Ultrasound will usually be used to see the fetus and the placenta during amniocentesis, chorionic villus sampling, and fetal blood sampling procedures.

To assess the growth of the fetus

If, by measuring your abdomen, your doctor feels that the fetus may not be growing as much as it should or is growing too rapidly, he or she may do an ultrasound scan. A second scan, performed 3 or 4 weeks later, can assess the rate at which the fetus is growing.

To detect a multiple pregnancy

If your doctor suspects you may be carrying more than one fetus, an ultrasound scan may be done to determine how many fetuses are present.

To detect fetal abnormalities

Ultrasound can help identify some developmental abnormalities in the fetus. Ultrasound can also identify the sex of the fetus, which may be important information if there is a family history of an inherited condition that usually affects only boys (such as Duchenne type muscular dystrophy). Parents may want to have additional testing done if they are considering terminating the pregnancy.

How ultrasound is performed

A device called a transducer is moved along the surface of your abdomen. (In the very early stages of pregnancy, a transducer that is inserted into the vagina may be used to see the fetus more clearly.) Sound waves emitted by the transducer enter your body and are reflected back from your internal organs and the fetus. These sound waves are translated into an image on a computer screen.

Fetal blood sampling

A blood sample from the fetus's umbilical cord can be taken and tested to determine if the fetus has become anemic or to detect some inherited disorders. Under the guidance of ultrasound, blood is withdrawn through a needle that is inserted into a blood vessel in the umbilical cord.

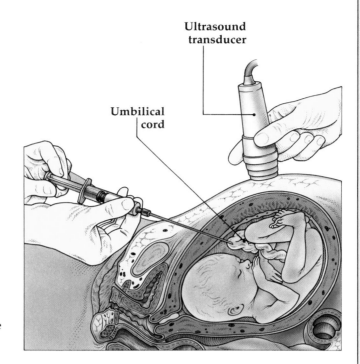

Ultrasound transducer

Umbilical cord

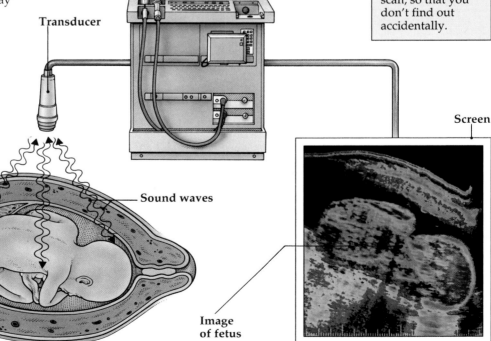

Computer

Transducer

Sound waves

Image of fetus

Screen

A BOY OR GIRL?

Ultrasound scanning is an optional test – not a routine part of prenatal care – and should not be performed solely to determine the sex of your baby. But, because ultrasound scanning is appropriate in a variety of special circumstances, it is quite common. If you have an ultrasound scan at 18 weeks or later, the scan may reveal (depending on the position of the fetus during the scan) whether you are going to have a boy or a girl. Some couples want to know – others want to be surprised at the time the baby is born. If you do not want to know the sex of your baby, be sure to tell your doctor or the technician doing the scan, so that you don't find out accidentally.

GOOD HEALTH DURING PREGNANCY

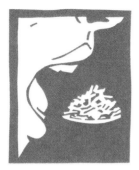

T AKING CARE OF YOURSELF during pregnancy is important to your health and the health of your baby. You can do a great deal to give your baby the best possible start in life, such as eating well, getting plenty of rest, and exercising regularly. Being pregnant may require changing or adding to your everyday health routines.

A balanced diet is an essential part of taking good care of yourself during your pregnancy. Eating a variety of healthy foods provides you and the developing fetus with adequate protein, vitamins, minerals, and other nutrients. But remember, eating well does not mean overeating and gaining too much weight.

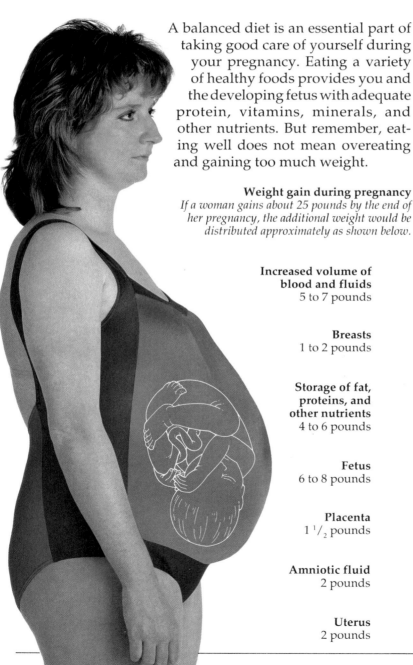

Weight gain during pregnancy
If a woman gains about 25 pounds by the end of her pregnancy, the additional weight would be distributed approximately as shown below.

Increased volume of blood and fluids
5 to 7 pounds

Breasts
1 to 2 pounds

Storage of fat, proteins, and other nutrients
4 to 6 pounds

Fetus
6 to 8 pounds

Placenta
1 1/2 pounds

Amniotic fluid
2 pounds

Uterus
2 pounds

EATING WISELY

Gaining a reasonable amount of weight during pregnancy helps your body nourish the fetus. Most women gain about 25 to 30 pounds. Talk to your doctor about the best weight gain for you.

During pregnancy, your rate of metabolism increases, which means you use up energy from food (in the form of calories) faster. Most pregnant women should increase their calorie intake by 300 calories a day. The increased calories are needed for growth of the fetus and placenta as well as the growth and changes in your body tissues.

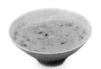

Yogurt (8 ounces)
7.7 grams of protein

Dried peas or beans (2 ounces)
15 grams of protein

Eggs (1 large)
6.5 grams of protein

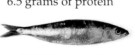

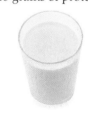

Fish (4 ounces)
34 grams of protein

Milk (32 ounces)
41.3 grams of protein

Protein
Throughout your pregnancy, you need an additional 10 to 15 grams of protein beyond the normal daily requirement of 45 grams. Foods high in protein are eggs, milk and milk products, lean meat, poultry, fish, and dried peas or beans.

A well-balanced diet

The healthy foods you eat help the fetus grow and develop. Eat a well-balanced diet every day, choosing a variety of foods, including fruits and vegetables, whole-grain products, protein foods, and milk and milk products.

Fats provide extra calories and are high in vitamins A and D. Keep your fat intake at no more than 30 percent of your total calories, and eat mainly unsaturated fats, such as those in most vegetable oils and some soft margarines. Check food labels carefully.

Foods such as brown rice and whole-grain bread are high in unrefined carbohydrates and are good sources of vitamins, minerals, and fiber. Sweets, which contain carbohydrates in the form of refined starch and sugar, have little nutritional value and are low in fiber.

Vitamins and minerals

A well-balanced diet usually provides adequate amounts of most vitamins, minerals, and nutrients during pregnancy, but talk to your doctor about the need for additional vitamin and mineral supplements. Some women develop a deficiency in the minerals iron and calcium – particularly during the last trimester, when the needs of the fetus are greatest. Some foods rich in essential minerals are shown below and at right.

Your body needs an increased amount of the vitamin folic acid to make nucleic acids, which are essential for rapidly dividing cells. Because your body cannot store folic acid, doctors recommend consuming 0.4 milligrams of folic acid daily during pregnancy. Foods high in folic acid are organ meats, green leafy vegetables, nuts, and whole-grain bread.

Dried fruits (2 ounces)
2 milligrams of iron

Whole-grain bread (2 slices)
1.4 milligrams of iron

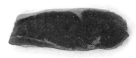

Sirloin steak (8 ounces)
5.6 milligrams of iron

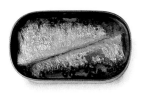

Sardines (4 ounces)
400 milligrams of calcium

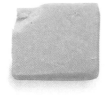

Cheese (1 ounce)
200 milligrams of calcium

Walnuts (3 ounces)
2 milligrams of zinc

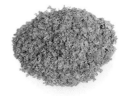

Wheat germ (1 ounce)
4.7 milligrams of zinc

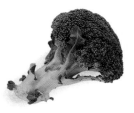

Broccoli (4 ounces)
0.9 milligrams of iron

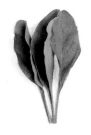

Spinach (4 ounces)
105 milligrams of calcium

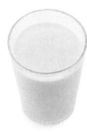

Milk (32 ounces)
720 milligrams of calcium

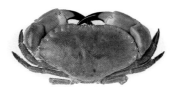

Crab (2 ounces)
2.5 milligrams of zinc

Eggs (1 large)
0.7 milligrams of zinc

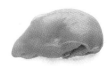

Chicken (4 ounces)
1.5 milligrams of iron

Calcium
Calcium is essential for the development of the fetus's teeth and bones. During pregnancy, you need about 1,200 milligrams of calcium a day. Foods high in calcium are milk, cheese, green leafy vegetables, and canned fish such as sardines. Your intake of calcium-rich foods should include 1 quart of low-fat milk each day. Milk is also high in vitamin D, which your body needs to absorb calcium.

Zinc
Your body needs zinc for growth and energy production. During pregnancy, the recommended daily requirement of zinc is 20 milligrams. Foods high in zinc include seafood, whole-grain cereals, meats, eggs, milk, nuts, and wheat germ.

Iron
As the volume of your blood increases during pregnancy, you need up to 30 milligrams of iron a day to manufacture the hemoglobin (the oxygen-carrying substance in red blood cells) needed for the increased number of red blood cells. Foods rich in iron are red meat, liver, shellfish, poultry, some vegetables, dried fruits, and whole-grain bread.

FIBER AND FLUIDS

Fiber and fluids play a vital role in your digestive process. Eating a high-fiber diet and drinking plenty of fluids help encourage the efficient passage of stools through the bowels and can help prevent constipation.

High-fiber foods
Your diet should contain between 20 and 30 grams of fiber a day. A selection of foods high in fiber is shown below.

Almonds
(2 ounces)
8 grams of fiber

Dried apricots
(2 ounces)
14 grams of fiber

Peas
(4 ounces)
8 grams of fiber

Bananas
(7 ounces)
3.5 grams of fiber

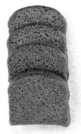

Whole-grain bread
(4 slices)
8 grams of fiber

Bran
(¹/₂ tablespoon)
3 grams of fiber

Drink plenty of fluids
It is especially important to drink plenty of fluids during your pregnancy to help keep your kidneys working efficiently and to help prevent constipation. You should drink at least six to eight glasses of fluids every day.

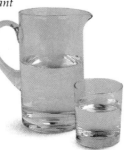

The need for other vitamins, such as vitamins B and C, also increases during pregnancy. Vitamin B_6 is essential for the development of the fetus's nervous system; the recommended daily requirement during pregnancy is 2.5 milligrams. Foods rich in vitamin B_6 include organ meats, fish, poultry, whole-grain products, potatoes, and bananas. Vitamin B_{12} is needed for the production of red blood cells and the development of the fetus's nervous system. Although vitamin B_{12} deficiency is rare during pregnancy (except among women on a strict vegetarian diet), some doctors advise increasing the recommended daily requirement of 2 micrograms to 3 micrograms. Foods high in vitamin B_{12} include fish, milk, liver, and fortified breakfast cereals. Be sure your diet includes foods rich in vitamin C every day, because vitamin C cannot be stored in the body (see below).

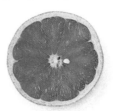

¹/₂ grapefruit
(6 ounces)
37 milligrams
of vitamin C

Green peppers
(4 ounces)
145 milligrams
of vitamin C

Strawberries
(4 ounces)
67 milligrams
of vitamin C

Vitamin C
Vitamin C is essential for the growth of the fetus and the development of strong bones and teeth. During pregnancy, the recommended daily requirement of vitamin C is 80 milligrams. Fresh fruit and vegetables are good sources of vitamin C.

Vegetarian diet

A well-planned vegetarian diet that includes cheese, milk, eggs, cereals, nuts, vegetables, and fruit can be an adequate diet for a healthy pregnancy. If you are on a vegetarian diet, check with your doctor to be sure that you are getting all the nutrients you need.

HEALTHY HABITS

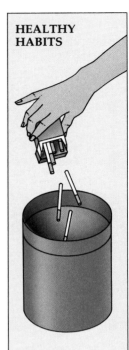

◆ Smoking is not only harmful to you, but to the fetus as well. If you did not stop smoking before you became pregnant, stop now.

◆ There is no safe level of alcohol consumption during pregnancy. Do not drink any alcoholic beverages while you are pregnant.

◆ Try to avoid caffeine – too much caffeine may increase the fetus's heart rate.

◆ Your body needs only a moderate amount of salt – don't overdo it.

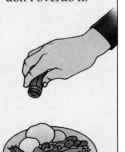

DRUGS DURING PREGNANCY

Do not take any drugs or medications during pregnancy without first consulting your doctor. Potentially dangerous drugs include not only drugs of abuse but also prescription drugs and many medications that you can buy over the counter. If you take medication for a medical condition such as hypertension or epilepsy, you should consult your doctor before you try to become pregnant, so that any changes in your medication can be made if necessary. Use of some medications should not be stopped suddenly. The table below explains the potential dangers some medications pose to a pregnant woman and the fetus, but these risks are often much lower than the risks of stopping treatment.

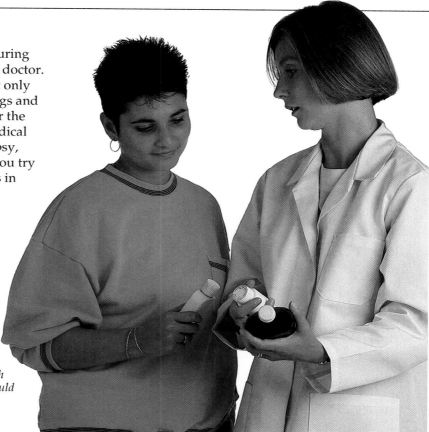

Over-the-counter drugs during pregnancy
Check with your doctor before you take any drugs during pregnancy. Even such items as cough syrup and painkillers could have an effect on the fetus.

Angiotensin-converting enzyme (ACE) inhibitors
Prescribed for high blood pressure.
ACE inhibitors taken during the middle or late stages of pregnancy may have serious adverse effects on the fetus – low blood pressure, kidney problems, birth defects, or even death.

Anticoagulants
Prescribed to prevent formation of blood clots or to prevent enlargement of existing blood clots.
Although heparin is relatively safe when taken during pregnancy, it may cause excessive bleeding during delivery. Warfarin may cause malformation of the fetus if this drug is taken during the early stages of pregnancy. If warfarin is taken near the time of delivery, it may cause excessive bleeding during childbirth.

Anticonvulsants
Prescribed primarily to prevent epileptic seizures.
Anticonvulsants can cause malformation of the fetus. The risk is greater if more than one anticonvulsant drug has been prescribed. If carbamazepine and ethosuximide are taken during the first trimester of pregnancy, they may cause neural tube defects such as spina bifida (failure of the bones of the spine to close). Phenobarbital, phenytoin, and valproic acid may cause malformation of the fetus, damage to the fetus's liver, or internal bleeding in the baby at birth.

Tetracyclines
A group of antibiotics prescribed for infections.
Tetracyclines may affect development of the fetus's bones and teeth and cause permanent discoloration of a child's teeth.

Aspirin and other nonsteroidal anti-inflammatory drugs (NSAIDs)
Prescribed primarily for relieving pain, stiffness, and inflammation and for reducing fever.
Aspirin (and possibly other NSAIDs) can affect the fetus's blood-clotting mechanism, cause lung damage and pulmonary hypertension (increased blood pressure in the arteries supplying the lungs), and adversely affect liver function. These drugs may also have adverse effects on the pregnant woman, including prolonging the length of pregnancy, increasing the duration of labor, and causing excessive bleeding during delivery.

Beta blockers
Prescribed for high blood pressure, angina, heart rhythm disturbances, and hand tremors.
Beta blockers may slow the growth of the fetus and can cause a slow heart rate, low blood pressure, and a low level of blood glucose (a sugar) in the newborn baby.

Isotretinoin
Prescribed for acne and other skin disorders.
Isotretinoin is likely to cause severe deformities of the fetus (even if the fetus is exposed to the drug for only a short time) and increases a woman's risk of miscarriage.

Sulfonamides
A group of antibacterial drugs prescribed for urinary tract, eye, ear, skin, and respiratory infections.
Sulfonamide antibiotics can adversely affect the fetus's liver function (which may lead to brain damage) and can cause blood disorders in the fetus.

Changes in your gums
The increased level of the hormone progesterone during pregnancy makes your gums soft and spongy, allowing bacteria to flourish more easily between your teeth and gums. In some women, a swelling develops (see below). This swelling often disappears without treatment after delivery.

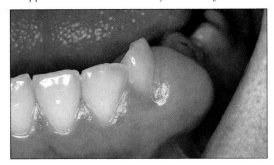

Dental care

Your teeth and gums may be more susceptible to infection while you are pregnant (see above). Common discomforts of pregnancy may affect your oral hygiene habits. For example, putting a toothbrush toward the back of the mouth sometimes triggers vomiting in women who are experiencing morning sickness.

Be sure to have regular dental cleanings and check-ups throughout your pregnancy. When you visit your dentist, tell him or her that you are pregnant, particularly if X-rays are needed. Your dentist will schedule treatment based on the urgency of the treatment needed and the stage of your pregnancy. Local anesthetics can be safely used for dental procedures during pregnancy.

X-rays during pregnancy

A woman who is pregnant or trying to conceive should not have an X-ray unless it is essential and cannot be postponed. X-rays are potentially harmful to the fetus and may increase the risk of leukemia or other types of cancer in childhood. The risk of X-rays harming the fetus is highest in the first trimester.

If an X-ray is necessary and you are pregnant or think you might be pregnant, be sure to tell the X-ray technician or the doctor. During the X-ray, the lead shield that is placed over your abdomen helps protect the fetus.

Video display terminals
Studies have shown that use of video display terminals during pregnancy poses no detectable radiation hazard related to miscarriage and birth defects. The radiation levels emitted from video display terminals are well below current occupational safety standards. However, unproven concerns about possible risks remain, and scientific debate and research continue.

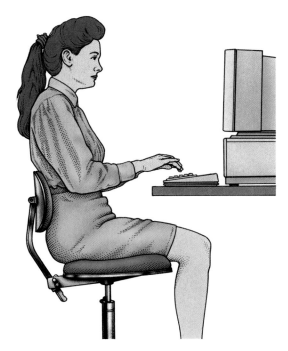

Flat or inverted nipples
If your nipples are flat or inverted, you may want to talk to your doctor about wearing nipple shields under your bra. The shields gently pull your nipples outward so that breast-feeding will be easier. The shields are usually worn for a few hours every day from week 15 of pregnancy.

Sex during pregnancy

Sexual intercourse can usually be continued throughout your pregnancy without risk to the fetus. The fetus is well protected inside the amniotic sac and the opening to the uterus is sealed by a plug of mucus. As your pregnancy progresses, you and your partner should avoid putting weight directly on your abdomen during sexual intercourse.

Preparing for breast-feeding

If you are planning to breast-feed your baby, you should start preparing your nipples during the last month of your pregnancy to help prevent nursing problems. Wear a well-fitting bra to help your muscles support the increased weight of your breasts. Exposing your nipples to air and light whenever possible helps toughen them. Talk to your doctor about techniques you can use to make your nipples easier for your baby to grasp.

TRAVEL

Traveling long distances can be stressful when you are pregnant, especially during the last 3 months. Always consult your doctor if you plan to travel. Here are some helpful tips to make your trip more comfortable and relaxing.

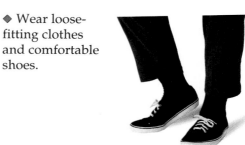

◆ Try to plan your trip so that you have plenty of time to relax and rest.

◆ If you are traveling a long way from home, your doctor may be able to refer you to a doctor in the area. If this isn't possible, be sure to get the telephone number and address of the nearest hospital in case of an emergency.

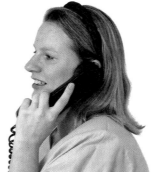

Airline travel
Always check with your doctor before scheduling airline travel. Also check with the airline; some airlines have regulations about pregnant women. During your flight, get up and stretch your legs once an hour. Sitting for long periods can lead to swelling and cramps in your legs.

◆ Wear loose-fitting clothes and comfortable shoes.

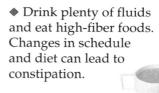

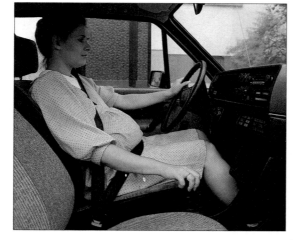

How to adjust your seat belt
Fasten the lap belt as low as possible across your abdomen. Place the shoulder strap across the center of your chest.

◆ Take extra cushions or pillows to place behind your back or neck.

◆ Drink plenty of fluids and eat high-fiber foods. Changes in schedule and diet can lead to constipation.

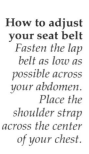

Preparing your children

If you have children, talk to them about the new baby and the special things that older brothers and sisters can do. Try to include the children in your preparations to bring the baby home – for example, take the children with you when you shop for the new baby or let them help decorate the baby's room. Explain to your children any arrangements you have made with a friend or relative to care for them when it is time to deliver the baby.

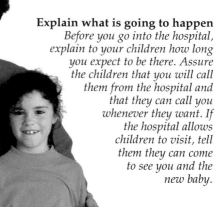

Explain what is going to happen
Before you go into the hospital, explain to your children how long you expect to be there. Assure the children that you will call them from the hospital and that they can call you whenever they want. If the hospital allows children to visit, tell them they can come to see you and the new baby.

EXERCISE DURING PREGNANCY

Exercising regularly during pregnancy will help you to control your weight, will prepare you for the physical demands of labor and delivery, and will help you to recover more quickly from the strain of childbirth. Exercise can also help reduce or eliminate some of the minor discomforts that you may experience, such as constipation and backache.

EXERCISE TIPS

◆ Do warm-up and cool-down exercises before and after exercising.
◆ Stop exercising as soon as you feel tired or out of breath.
◆ Drink plenty of fluids before and after exercising to avoid dehydration.
◆ Wear loose-fitting layers of clothing that can be removed as you warm up, a support bra, and comfortable shoes that support your feet and ankles.

Talk to your doctor about an exercise program that is right for you. Some exercise classes are designed especially for pregnant women. If you are accustomed to energetic exercise, such as jogging or playing tennis, you can usually continue this type of exercise while you are pregnant, so long as you feel comfortable. Pregnancy is not the time to begin a strenuous exercise program; start with a modest amount of exercise and gradually increase the amount every day.

WARNING

Consult your doctor before beginning an exercise program, especially if you are expecting twins or have any of the following:
◆ Anemia
◆ Diabetes
◆ Heart palpitations
◆ Hypertension
◆ History of bleeding
◆ Low body weight
◆ Obesity
◆ Thyroid problems
◆ History of premature labor, miscarriage, or other problems during pregnancy

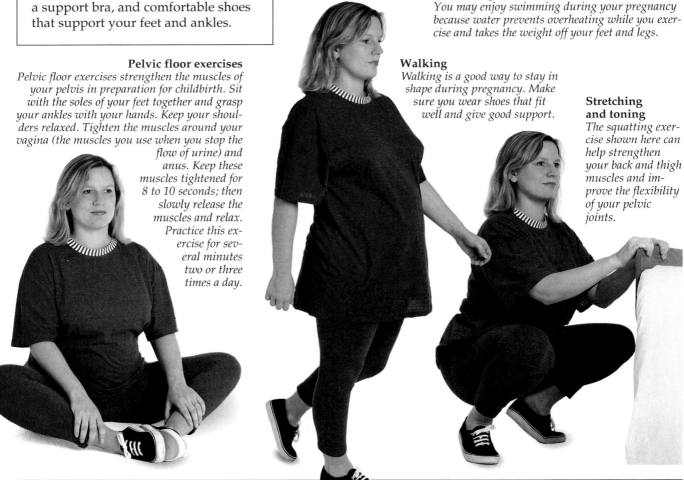

Swimming
You may enjoy swimming during your pregnancy because water prevents overheating while you exercise and takes the weight off your feet and legs.

Walking
Walking is a good way to stay in shape during pregnancy. Make sure you wear shoes that fit well and give good support.

Stretching and toning
The squatting exercise shown here can help strengthen your back and thigh muscles and improve the flexibility of your pelvic joints.

Pelvic floor exercises
Pelvic floor exercises strengthen the muscles of your pelvis in preparation for childbirth. Sit with the soles of your feet together and grasp your ankles with your hands. Keep your shoulders relaxed. Tighten the muscles around your vagina (the muscles you use when you stop the flow of urine) and anus. Keep these muscles tightened for 8 to 10 seconds; then slowly release the muscles and relax. Practice this exercise for several minutes two or three times a day.

CHILDBIRTH EDUCATION CLASSES

Childbirth education classes help prepare parents-to-be by teaching them about pregnancy and childbirth. The focus and scope of these classes differ. The topics covered may include prenatal care, how pregnancy progresses, the process of labor and delivery, methods of childbirth, and how to care for your newborn baby.

If you take a childbirth education class, be sure to choose one that is recommended by your health care professional so that there are no conflicts about methods and philosophies. Some classes teach a structured method of childbirth, while others concentrate more on understanding and responding to the body's sensations and needs. For example, the Lamaze method teaches relaxation techniques and physical conditioning, with the main emphasis on directed patterns of breathing that are very active and rapid. The Bradley approach includes instruction on the importance of good health and nutrition during pregnancy. It teaches physical conditioning exercises, with emphasis on slow, deep breathing and deep relaxation.

A team effort
The emphasis of childbirth education classes is to develop a working and supportive team effort by the woman, her partner, and the health care professional. Childbirth education classes will provide you with an opportunity to share experiences, ask questions, and practice breathing and relaxation techniques.

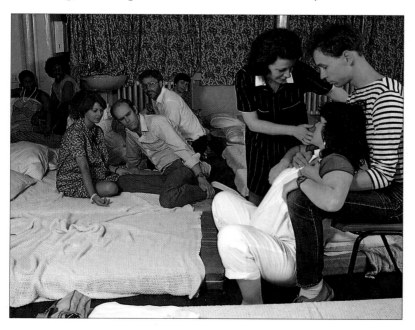

ASK YOUR DOCTOR
TAKING CARE OF YOURSELF

Q **Before I knew I was pregnant I drank a couple of glasses of wine at a party. The following week I found out I was pregnant and have not had any alcohol since that party. I know that drinking alcohol is dangerous during pregnancy. Have I harmed my baby?**

A Probably not. The critical time when the developing fetus might be harmed by drinking alcohol is between week 6 and week 12. But, because there is no established safe level for consumption of alcohol during pregnancy, it is important to abstain from alcohol throughout the rest of your pregnancy.

Q **How long is it safe for me to continue working now that I am expecting a baby?**

A Talk to your doctor to determine how long you should continue working. Many doctors believe that you should stop working by the 38th week of pregnancy. As long as you are in good health, there is no reason why you should not continue to work, providing that the type of work you do cannot put either you or your baby at risk.

Q **Before I became pregnant, I used to enjoy the sauna and the steam room. Is it safe for me to continue these activities now that I am pregnant?**

A Probably not. Saunas, steam rooms, hot tubs, or even very hot baths can increase your body temperature above 102°F, which could be hazardous to the development of the fetus, especially in the early months of pregnancy.

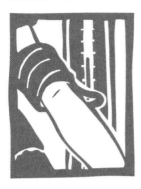

PREGNANCY DISORDERS

MOST WOMEN HAVE normal, healthy pregnancies. Although pregnancy may sometimes cause minor discomforts, most of the problems that can arise are not serious. However, some disorders that may occur can be a threat to you and/or the developing fetus. You need to be alert to the possible warning signs of problems that require medical attention. Consult your doctor if you are concerned or are not sure what certain symptoms mean.

Some disorders can develop soon after conception and may prevent the pregnancy from progressing normally. Other disorders can be treated and the pregnancy can continue.

EARLY PROBLEMS

A pregnant woman who experiences vaginal bleeding at any time during pregnancy should consult her doctor immediately, because bleeding can be an early indication of a miscarriage (see page 84). In some cases, a miscarriage in the very early stages of pregnancy may resemble a heavy menstrual period. In about one of every five pregnancies, a miscarriage occurs in the first trimester, usually as a result of a chromosome abnormality in the embryo.

Occasionally, the fertilized egg fails to implant itself in the lining of the uterus but implants elsewhere in the abdomen, usually in a fallopian tube. This is called an ectopic pregnancy (see page 86). An ectopic pregnancy causes severe abdominal pain and requires immediate surgery to remove the embryo.

Hydatidiform mole

A hydatidiform mole is a rare, noncancerous tumor that may form from placental tissue in which an embryo failed to develop. The tumor produces large amounts of the hormone human chorionic gonadotropin, which may cause severe nausea and vomiting. The tumor is removed by suctioning out the contents of the uterus. Women who have had such a tumor removed should have follow-up examinations and blood tests for at least a year because there is a slight risk that a cancerous tumor may develop.

A rare tumor
A hydatidiform mole is a rare tumor that develops from placental tissue. Resembling a bunch of grapes, a hydatidiform mole can be diagnosed by ultrasound scanning and by blood and urine tests, which detect the high levels of human chorionic gonadotropin produced by the tumor.

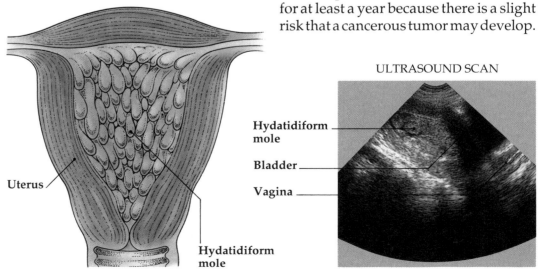

Uterus

Hydatidiform mole

ULTRASOUND SCAN

Hydatidiform mole

Bladder

Vagina

PREECLAMPSIA AND ECLAMPSIA

Preeclampsia is a serious condition in which the woman's blood pressure gradually rises to an abnormal level. This condition can develop during the second half of pregnancy. A woman with preeclampsia will also have edema (accumulation of fluid in body tissues). Untreated, preeclampsia can lead to eclampsia, a condition that causes the woman to have seizures that can be fatal to her and/or the fetus.

The cause of preeclampsia is unknown. One theory is that the condition results from the woman's immune system reacting abnormally to the presence of the fetus, leading to the release of chemicals that cause the woman's blood vessels to narrow. This narrowing of the vessels raises her blood pressure. Preeclampsia develops most often in a first pregnancy and is more likely to occur if a woman has a history of diabetes, high blood pressure, or kidney disease.

Women with preeclampsia are often admitted to the hospital for evaluation and treatment. Mild preeclampsia may be treated by resting in bed and restricting dietary intake of sodium. Medications to lower blood pressure may

Urine test for preeclampsia
If your doctor suspects that you have preeclampsia, he or she may order a urine test. The technician dips a chemically coated stick into a sample of your urine. A change in color indicates the presence of protein in the urine, which is one of the signs of preeclampsia.

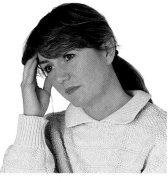

Warning signs
Symptoms of preeclampsia include persistent, severe headache, sudden weight gain, nausea, vomiting, abdominal pain, and blurred vision.

What are fibroids?
A fibroid is a noncancerous tumor, consisting of muscle and connective tissue, that grows within the wall of the uterus. Your doctor may suspect fibroids if the uterus appears to be too large for the stage of your pregnancy. He or she may be able to feel a firm, irregular lump through your abdominal wall.

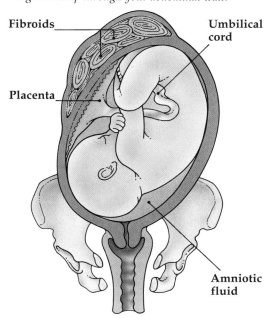

Fibroids

Umbilical cord

Placenta

Amniotic fluid

also be given. These treatments may temporarily improve the condition. However, if your blood pressure continues to rise and severe preeclampsia develops, your doctor may decide to induce labor, because the only "cure" for preeclampsia is to end the pregnancy.

FIBROIDS

Fibroids are noncancerous tumors of the muscles in the uterus. These tumors are the most commonly occurring type of tumor in women over 30 and develop in about 7 percent of pregnant women.

In many cases, fibroids do not cause symptoms, especially if they are small. Most pregnant women with fibroids deliver without any problems. But large fibroids – depending on their position in the uterus – can obstruct passage of the baby during delivery; in some cases a cesarean section is necessary. Fibroids often shrink after delivery and may require no further treatment.

PLACENTAL DISORDERS

One of the most crucial factors in the development of the fetus is a healthy placenta. The placenta forms the vital link between your body and the fetus's body.

PLACENTA PREVIA

In placenta previa, the placenta is implanted abnormally low in the uterus. The cause is unknown, although the size, contour, and tissue texture of the uterus may play a role. Placenta previa occurs more often among women who have had several children and women having twins. The severity of this disorder depends on the position of the placenta. Placenta previa may not affect the pregnancy but, in severe cases, it may prevent the placenta from functioning normally and can lead to premature labor, severe vaginal bleeding during pregnancy or at delivery, and obstruction of the opening of the cervix at delivery.

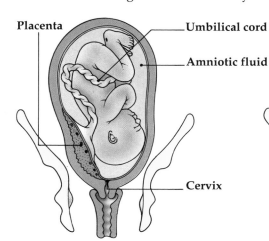

Marginal placenta previa
The placenta is implanted near the opening of the cervix.

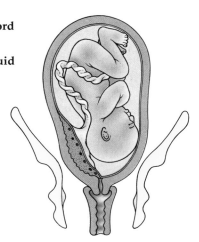

Partial placenta previa
The placenta covers only a portion of the opening of the cervix.

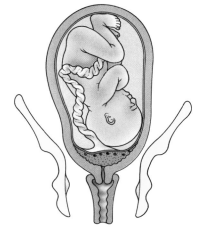

Complete placenta previa
The placenta covers the entire opening of the cervix.

TREATING PLACENTAL DISORDERS

Bleeding caused by placental disorders requires immediate medical care. If your delivery date is more than 3 weeks away and the bleeding is slight, it may stop with bed rest; if the bleeding recurs, you may need to rest in bed for the rest of your pregnancy. If bleeding persists or you are more than 37 weeks' pregnant, your doctor may deliver your baby immediately.

PLACENTAL ABRUPTION

In placental abruption, part of a normally positioned placenta becomes detached from the wall of the uterus. The cause is unknown, although some doctors believe placental abruption may be related to a deficiency of the vitamin folic acid. Placental abruption is more common in women with high blood pressure. Detachment of the placenta usually causes sudden abdominal pain. Bleeding is not always apparent, because the blood is sometimes retained between the placenta and the wall of the uterus. Placental abruption may cause a life-threatening loss of blood, may prevent the placenta from functioning normally, and may lead to premature labor.

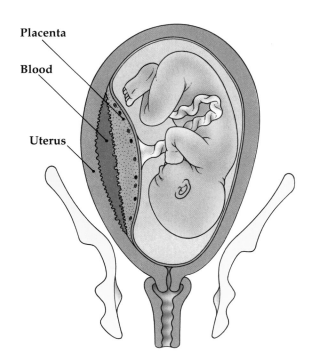

DISORDERS OF THE AMNIOTIC FLUID

Amniotic fluid surrounds and protects the fetus (see page 31). The fluid is contained within a membrane called the amniotic sac. The volume of amniotic fluid increases up until weeks 36 to 38 and then begins to decrease. Your doctor will assess the volume of the amniotic fluid at each prenatal visit by feeling and measuring your abdomen (and, in some cases, by doing an ultrasound scan).

Too much amniotic fluid

An excess amount of amniotic fluid is known as polyhydramnios. Excess amniotic fluid may build up gradually or accumulate quickly. Symptoms of polyhydramnios are an abdominal size that is larger than expected for the length of the pregnancy, abdominal discomfort, and occasionally breathlessness, nausea, or swelling of the legs.

If polyhydramnios occurs, tests may be done to check for fetal abnormalities. In most cases, the fetus is normal and the polyhydramnios does not require treatment. Occasionally, some of the fluid is withdrawn to relieve symptoms, using a procedure similar to amniocentesis. If symptoms occur in late pregnancy and are severe, your doctor may induce labor.

Too little amniotic fluid

An abnormally small amount of amniotic fluid is called oligohydramnios. It may be a sign that the woman has severe preeclampsia (see page 69) or may indicate kidney or urinary abnormalities in the fetus. If the oligohydramnios occurs early in pregnancy, it can cause a miscarriage. If it occurs during the late stages of pregnancy, it can result in deformity of the fetus or even fetal death.

If oligohydramnios is suspected, the doctor will try to treat the disorder that has caused this condition. If you are more than 37 weeks' pregnant, your doctor may induce labor.

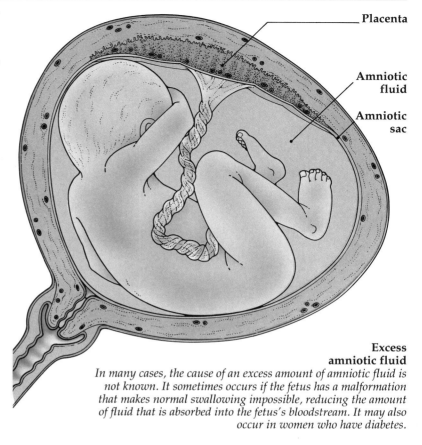

Placenta

Amniotic fluid

Amniotic sac

Excess amniotic fluid
In many cases, the cause of an excess amount of amniotic fluid is not known. It sometimes occurs if the fetus has a malformation that makes normal swallowing impossible, reducing the amount of fluid that is absorbed into the fetus's bloodstream. It may also occur in women who have diabetes.

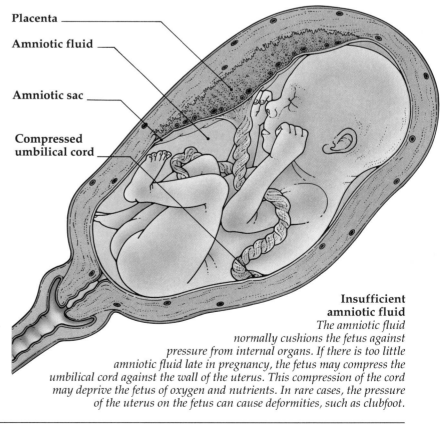

Placenta

Amniotic fluid

Amniotic sac

Compressed umbilical cord

Insufficient amniotic fluid
The amniotic fluid normally cushions the fetus against pressure from internal organs. If there is too little amniotic fluid late in pregnancy, the fetus may compress the umbilical cord against the wall of the uterus. This compression of the cord may deprive the fetus of oxygen and nutrients. In rare cases, the pressure of the uterus on the fetus can cause deformities, such as clubfoot.

POOR FETAL GROWTH

Poor fetal growth means that the fetus is much smaller than expected for the stage of the pregnancy. Such babies may need special care after delivery.

Poor fetal growth has many causes. It may result from a chromosome defect or an infection passed on from the woman. More often, poor fetal growth is caused by inadequate nutrition provided by the placenta, a condition known as placental insufficiency. Placental insufficiency can be the result of a placental disorder (see page 70) or may be caused by a multiple pregnancy (two or more fetuses), smoking, drinking alcohol, or high blood pressure or other medical conditions. In some cases, the cause of placental insufficiency is never found.

Your doctor may suspect poor fetal growth if your uterus is smaller than expected for the length of pregnancy (see THE INCREASING SIZE OF THE UTERUS on page 38). An ultrasound scan and blood tests are often used to help make a diagnosis. If poor fetal growth is diagnosed, the cause will be treated and your pregnancy will be carefully monitored.

PREMATURE RUPTURE OF MEMBRANES

Premature rupture of the membranes of the amniotic sac (which can occur anytime other than immediately before the onset of labor) can be dangerous to the woman and the fetus. Rupture often causes labor to start prematurely, can lead to infection, or may cause the umbilical cord to drop onto the cervix and be compressed by the fetus's head, which obstructs the oxygen supply to the fetus.

If you are less than 34 weeks' pregnant, your doctor may recommend bed rest to try to prolong your pregnancy so that the fetus can develop more before delivery. Some doctors give drugs to try to weaken or stop premature uterine contractions. After week 34, the fetus

Care of a premature baby
A premature baby is usually closely monitored in an incubator, where temperature and humidity are carefully controlled. A premature baby is at increased risk of injury during birth, breathing and liver problems, infection, a low blood sugar level, and anemia and has an increased tendency to bleed.

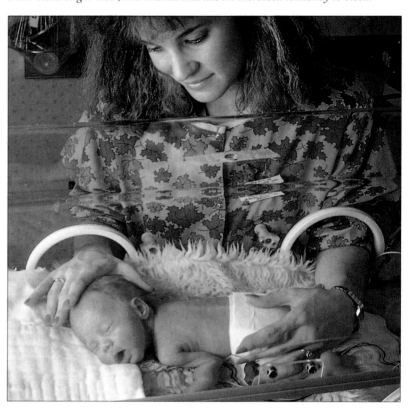

will probably be delivered because the risks of prolonging the pregnancy (such as infection) are greater than the risks to the fetus of premature birth.

PREMATURE LABOR

Labor is considered premature if it occurs before 37 weeks of pregnancy. About 9 percent of babies are born prematurely. Premature birth carries no risk for the mother, but a premature baby may not be sufficiently developed and may need to be put in an incubator. Causes of premature labor are preeclampsia, multiple pregnancy (two or more fetuses), placental abnormalities, infection in the uterus, or premature rupture of the membranes. In about 40 percent of cases, the cause is not known. Premature labor is more common in women who have had a previous premature delivery, in women under 20 or over 34 years old, in women who smoke, and in women who drink excessive amounts of alcohol during their pregnancy.

If you experience uterine contractions that occur every 10 minutes or more frequently and that do not stop within 30 to 60 minutes, call your doctor and go to the hospital immediately. If you are less than 34 weeks' pregnant, an attempt to stop premature labor is usually made by giving drugs that stop the contractions. After week 34 of pregnancy, labor may be allowed to continue.

ABNORMAL PRESENTATION

The presentation of the fetus describes the relationship of the fetus's body to that of the woman – for example, the fetus may be lying vertically or sideways. At term, more than 99 percent of fetuses

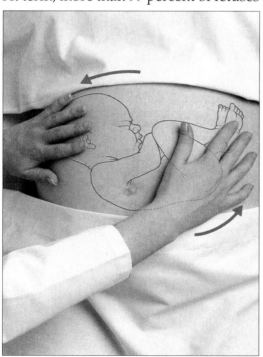

External version
If the fetus is in an abnormal presentation when it is time to deliver, your doctor may attempt to move the fetus into a longitudinal (vertical) presentation by manipulating it externally. This procedure is called external version. If external version is not successful, a cesarean section may be necessary.

Unstable presentation
In an unstable presentation, the fetus frequently changes its position in the uterus. If labor starts while the baby is lying sideways, complications can occur. For example, the umbilical cord may become compressed in the birth canal, cutting off the blood supply to the baby. A sideways presentation during labor requires a cesarean section to deliver the baby.

■■ Oblique (diagonal) presentation

■■ Longitudinal (vertical) presentation

■■ Transverse (sideways) presentation

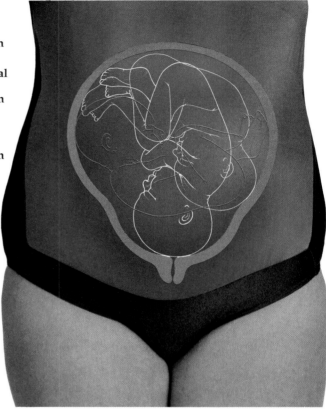

lie vertically in the woman's body. About 95 percent lie with their head down (called a cephalic presentation). Other fetuses present buttocks first (called a breech presentation – see page 104). Most fetuses settle into a vertical presentation from around the 32nd week onward.

Sometimes, the fetus keeps moving even after week 32 (called an unstable presentation). Unstable presentation occurs most commonly in women who have had many children, which reduces the tone and strength of the muscles in the uterus and abdominal wall. Other causes of an unstable presentation are excessive amniotic fluid or uterine abnormalities. In some cases, the fetus presents sideways (called a transverse presentation). A sideways presentation may be caused by fibroids or placenta previa.

FETAL HEAD POSITION

The fetus's neck is usually fully flexed forward so that the chin rests on his or her chest. This position allows the head to pass through the woman's pelvis. If the fetus's neck is not fully flexed, a cesarean section may be necessary (see page 112).

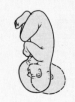

MONITOR YOUR SYMPTOMS
VAGINAL BLEEDING DURING PREGNANCY

If you notice any vaginal bleeding during your pregnancy, even only slight spotting, you should consult your doctor immediately. Vaginal bleeding may indicate a serious problem, but in many cases there is no danger to the pregnancy.

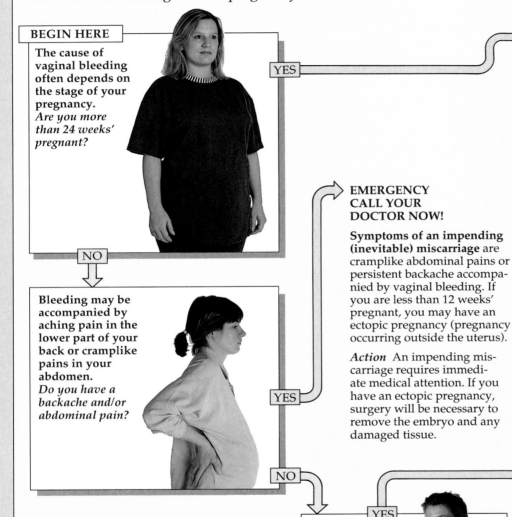

BEGIN HERE

The cause of vaginal bleeding often depends on the stage of your pregnancy. *Are you more than 24 weeks' pregnant?*

YES →

NO ↓

Bleeding may be accompanied by aching pain in the lower part of your back or cramplike pains in your abdomen. *Do you have a backache and/or abdominal pain?*

EMERGENCY CALL YOUR DOCTOR NOW!

Vaginal bleeding in the late stages of pregnancy may be caused by partial separation of the placenta from the wall of the uterus, by a placenta that is unusually low in the uterus, by bleeding from a vein in the vagina, or by abnormalities of the cervix. Spotting in the late stages of pregnancy can be caused by stretching of the cervix. Discharge of a blood-stained plug of mucus from the vagina may be the first sign of impending labor.

Action Often no treatment other than bed rest is needed to stop the bleeding. If bleeding is severe or continuous, it may be necessary to deliver the baby by inducing labor or by cesarean section.

EMERGENCY CALL YOUR DOCTOR NOW!

Symptoms of an impending (inevitable) miscarriage are cramplike abdominal pains or persistent backache accompanied by vaginal bleeding. If you are less than 12 weeks' pregnant, you may have an ectopic pregnancy (pregnancy occurring outside the uterus).

Action An impending miscarriage requires immediate medical attention. If you have an ectopic pregnancy, surgery will be necessary to remove the embryo and any damaged tissue.

YES

NO ↓

YES →

In the early stages of pregnancy, **spotting of blood** may occur at the time that your menstrual period would have been due. This spotting occurs because the placenta is not yet producing high enough levels of certain hormones to prevent slight shedding of the lining of the uterus.

Action Although spotting of blood usually poses no risk to the pregnancy, you should lie down and call your doctor. He or she will probably advise you to rest in bed until the bleeding stops.

Vaginal bleeding may occur in the early weeks of pregnancy. *Are you less than 14 weeks' pregnant?*

NO ←

EMERGENCY CALL YOUR DOCTOR NOW!

A threatened (possible) miscarriage is the usual diagnosis when vaginal bleeding occurs without pain in the middle stages of pregnancy. Bleeding may also be caused by an abnormality involving the cervix or inflammation of the vagina.

Action If a threatened miscarriage is diagnosed, your doctor may recommend that you decrease your level of activity, or possibly rest in bed. Other causes of vaginal bleeding can often be treated by your doctor.

CASE HISTORY
RISING BLOOD PRESSURE

JANET WAS EXPECTING **her first baby. She did not experience any problems, other than a short period of morning sickness and minor backaches, until week 32 of her pregnancy. One evening Janet noticed that her fingers were so swollen that she could no longer wear her wedding ring. At her regularly scheduled appointment the next day, Janet mentioned the swelling to her doctor.**

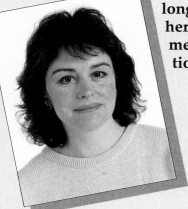

PERSONAL DETAILS
Name Janet Weinman
Age 34
Occupation Florist
Family Janet has no family history of any serious medical problem.

MEDICAL BACKGROUND
Janet has been in good health. Before she became pregnant, Janet saw her doctor only once a year to have checkups and a cervical (Pap) smear. During most of her pregnancy, Janet's blood pressure has been around 110/70.

THE CONSULTATION
Janet's doctor sees that her ankles as well as her fingers are swollen. He also finds that her blood pressure is higher than it was at her previous visit and that her weight has increased excessively. Results of a urine test show no abnormalities. The doctor arranges to see Janet again in a week and tells her to slow down her daily routine as much as possible and to get plenty of rest.

At Janet's next appointment, her blood pressure is 150/90. A urine test shows protein in her urine, which indicates her kidneys are not functioning completely normally. In addition to the swelling in her ankles and fingers, the tissues around her eyes have become puffy.

THE DIAGNOSIS
The doctor suspects that Janet has PREECLAMPSIA, a serious condition characterized by high blood pressure and retention of fluids that sometimes develops during pregnancy. The doctor arranges for Janet to be admitted to the hospital.

THE TREATMENT
In the hospital Janet must rest in bed. Her blood pressure and weight are monitored and blood and urine samples are tested to check her kidney function. An electronic instrument is placed on Janet's abdomen to monitor the fetus's heartbeat.

The next day, Janet's blood pressure has increased above 160/110. Her doctor instructs the nurses to give Janet a medication called hydralazine to try to lower her blood pressure. After several hours of intravenous medication, Janet's blood pressure remains high. Janet's doctor explains that, because the treatment has not lowered her high blood pressure, she could have a seizure, which would be life-threatening to both her and the baby. He tells her that the only way to lower her blood pressure is to deliver her baby.

OUTCOME
The doctor gives Janet oxytocin to induce labor and magnesium sulfate to prevent seizures. Janet delivers a small but healthy baby boy. He is carefully monitored in an incubator. Janet's blood pressure returns to normal and she is able to go home in a few days. The doctor reassures Janet that her son is doing fine and should be able to go home soon.

Visiting the baby
Janet and her husband are able to visit their son in the nursery. They are thrilled by reports of his progress every day and look forward with great anticipation to taking him home with them very soon.

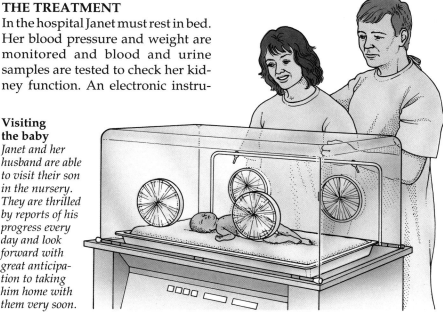

SERIOUS WARNING SIGNS DURING PREGNANCY

Most of the symptoms that a pregnant woman experiences are normal and result from the physical or hormonal changes that are occurring in her body. However, some symptoms may warn of a serious problem requiring immediate medical attention.

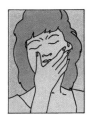

Excessive vomiting
Severe, persistent vomiting can lead to dehydration and disturbances in the body's normal chemical balance. It may be a sign of a multiple pregnancy (meaning there are two or more fetuses) or a hydatidiform mole (see page 68).

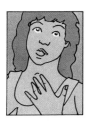

Sudden breathlessness
Sudden difficulty breathing could be a sign of a blood clot in the lungs (called a pulmonary embolism), a condition that can be life-threatening. During pregnancy, blood clots form more easily. Although this is your body's natural defense mechanism against bleeding after delivery, there is an increased risk of blood clots forming in the deep veins of the legs (called deep-vein thrombosis). Blood clots in the legs can become dislodged and move into the lungs.

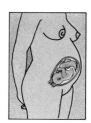

Decreased fetal movements
One important indicator of the fetus's well-being is its activity. Your doctor may suggest that you keep a "kick chart" (on which you note the movements of the fetus) from about the 30th week of your pregnancy. If you feel fewer than 10 fetal movements within a 12-hour period, call your doctor immediately.

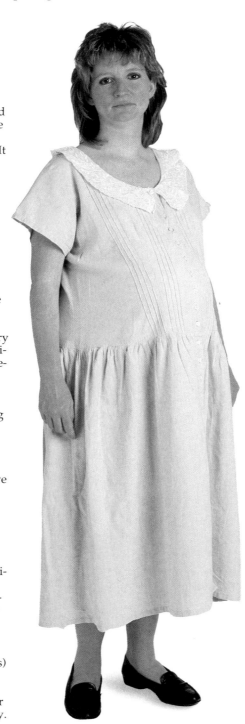

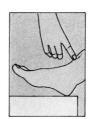

Severe swelling
Severe swelling in your feet, legs, and fingers as a result of excessive fluid that accumulates in these body tissues (called edema) could indicate preeclampsia (high blood pressure brought on by pregnancy) or heart failure if you have heart disease.

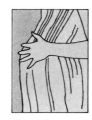

Severe, persistent, abdominal pain
Severe, persistent, abdominal pain – especially if accompanied by diarrhea, vomiting, drowsiness, confusion, or faintness – may be a sign of a serious disorder such as an ectopic pregnancy (a pregnancy that develops outside the uterus – usually in a fallopian tube), a miscarriage, or placental abruption (detachment of the placenta from the wall of the uterus). Abdominal pain can also indicate an illness that is unrelated to your pregnancy, such as appendicitis (inflammation of the appendix).

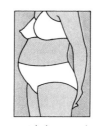

Vaginal bleeding
Painful bleeding before 20 weeks of pregnancy can be a sign of a miscarriage. If you are more than 20 weeks' pregnant, vaginal bleeding, whether or not it is associated with pain, may be caused by placenta previa (an abnormally positioned placenta) or placental abruption (detachment of the placenta from the wall of the uterus).

CASE HISTORY
WORRISOME BLEEDING

Cindy was delighted when a home pregnancy test indicated that she was pregnant again. She already had a 3-year-old son, who had been delivered normally after a healthy pregnancy. She visited her doctor, who confirmed her pregnancy with a urine test and a physical examination. At 14 weeks, Cindy experienced aching in the lower part of her back and noticed a small amount of blood on her underpants. Worried, Cindy called her doctor and had her husband take her to the clinic.

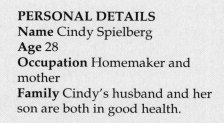

PERSONAL DETAILS
Name Cindy Spielberg
Age 28
Occupation Homemaker and mother
Family Cindy's husband and her son are both in good health.

MEDICAL BACKGROUND
Cindy is in good health, although she occasionally gets migraines. During her previous pregnancy, her headaches were not severe and she did not need to take any medication for her migraines.

THE CONSULTATION
Cindy tells her doctor about the bleeding and backache. The doctor examines Cindy's abdomen and feels that her uterus is soft and approximately the right size. He and Cindy listen to her baby's heartbeat using a technique called Doppler ultrasound. This type of ultrasound detects sound waves that are reflected off the fetus's heart. The reflected sound waves are converted into audible signals. The doctor also performs an internal (pelvic) examination. He notices mild bleeding from the cervix, which is still closed.

THE DIAGNOSIS
Cindy's doctor tells her that he is not absolutely certain of the cause of the bleeding. He thinks it might indicate a THREATENED MISCARRIAGE. He explains that the results of the Doppler ultrasound show the fetus's heartbeat is normal, and that the closed cervix indicates a miscarriage is not inevitable.

THE TREATMENT
The doctor tells Cindy that in many cases the cause of vaginal bleeding cannot be determined. He explains to her that the only treatment for a threatened miscarriage is bed rest, and reassures her by telling her that two thirds of women who experience a threatened miscarriage go on to deliver normal, healthy babies. After a week of bed rest, Cindy returns to see the doctor and tells him that she has not had any more bleeding. The doctor examines her and finds that the bleeding from the cervix has stopped. The doctor arranges for Cindy to have an ultrasound scan. The scan shows that the fetus is healthy and that the placenta is positioned normally in the uterus. The doctor tells Cindy to take things easy for a while and advises her and her husband to abstain from sexual intercourse for a few weeks.

THE OUTCOME
Cindy's pregnancy continues normally and 6 months later she gives birth to a healthy, 7 1/2 pound girl.

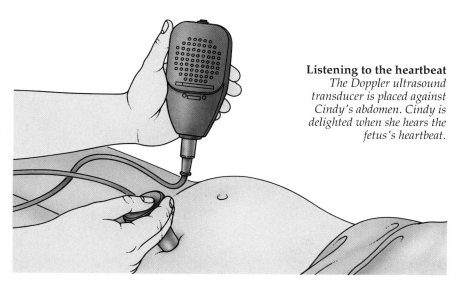

Listening to the heartbeat
The Doppler ultrasound transducer is placed against Cindy's abdomen. Cindy is delighted when she hears the fetus's heartbeat.

HIGH-RISK PREGNANCIES

A HIGH-RISK PREGNANCY is one in which there are factors that cause a woman to be at increased risk of experiencing problems. The greater risk of complications may be the result of the woman's age, a history of a genetic (inherited) disorder, problems during previous pregnancies, or a medical condition she had before she became pregnant. A woman who is pregnant with two or more fetuses is also considered to be at high risk.

Many problems that can occur during pregnancy can be predicted and then prevented or treated. Your medical history or the results of prenatal tests may indicate you are at an increased risk of complications. High-risk pregnancies require careful monitoring by your doctor. It is essential that you and your doctor work together to ensure the best possible outcome for your pregnancy.

TEENAGERS AND WOMEN OVER 35

In 1989, about 37 of every 1,000 girls aged 15 to 17 in the US had a baby. Teenage girls are often at increased risk of problems during pregnancy as a result of an unhealthy diet, use of alcohol and other drugs, having a sexually transmitted disease, and lack of prenatal care. Only one in five pregnant teenagers younger than 15 receives any prenatal care during the first 3 months of pregnancy. Many women today are delaying childbirth until their middle or late 30s. Every day an average of 100 women over 35 in the US give birth to their first child. Although a woman over 35 is considered to be at a somewhat increased risk of some problems during pregnancy (see PREGNANCY DISORDERS on page 68), most have uncomplicated pregnancies and deliver healthy babies.

BEING SERIOUSLY OVERWEIGHT

A woman who is seriously overweight when she becomes pregnant is at increased risk of developing preeclampsia (high blood pressure brought on by pregnancy) and gestational diabetes (diabetes during pregnancy). In addi-

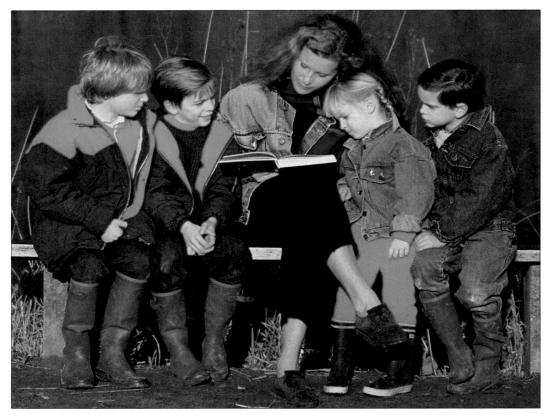

Effects of previous pregnancies
The muscles and ligaments of the uterus may become stretched and weakened after several pregnancies. As a result, the movements of the fetus can shift its position in the uterus more easily, which can lead to problems during labor and delivery (see UNSTABLE PRESENTATION on page 73).

tion, because seriously overweight women tend to have large babies, labor and delivery may be difficult. As a result, anesthesia and/or a cesarean section may be necessary, which increase the risks to both the woman and the fetus.

If you are overweight, it is best to try to lose weight before becoming pregnant. If you are pregnant and seriously over-weight, your doctor may recommend a diet that minimizes the amount of weight you gain during your pregnancy. He or she will monitor your diet to ensure it is providing all the essential nutrients for both you and the developing fetus.

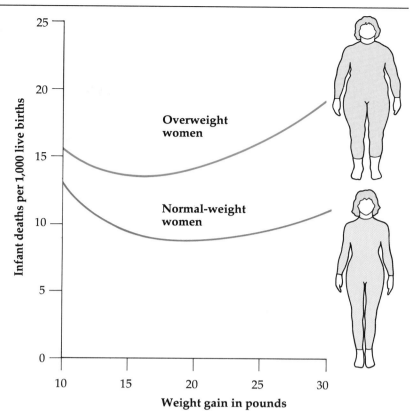

Increased death rates in infants born to overweight women
In overweight women, the rate of infant death increases significantly with the total amount of weight gained during pregnancy. The graph at right shows the numbers of infant deaths (per 1,000 live births) in the first 2 weeks of life as they relate to the amount of weight gained during pregnancy.

HOW THE Rh FACTOR CAN AFFECT PREGNANCY

Although the bloodstreams of the woman and the fetus are separate, blood cells from the fetus can cross the placenta and enter the woman's bloodstream. During delivery, some fetal blood cells always enter the woman's bloodstream. If a woman's blood group is Rh (Rhesus) negative and her partner's is Rh positive, the fetus's blood group may be Rh positive. As a result of the ex-change of blood cells, an Rh-negative woman's body may produce antibodies against the fetus's Rh-positive blood cells (called Rh sensitization). These antibodies break down the fetus's red blood cells, which may cause anemia in the fetus.

Preventing Rh sensitization
An injection of a blood product called Rh immu-noglobulin can be given to prevent sensitization. Rh immunoglobulin suppresses the ability of a woman's body to produce antibod-ies against Rh-positive red blood cells. The injection may be given to unsensitized Rh-nega-tive women during pregnancy and after delivery to prevent problems in future pregnancies.

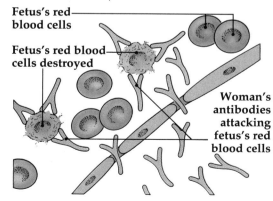

First Rh-positive fetus
A woman with Rh-negative blood may become "Rh sensitized" if the fetus has Rh-positive blood. This means the woman's body produces antibodies to fight the fetus's blood cells as if they were a harmful substance. During a woman's first pregnancy, the baby is usually born before a significant amount of these antibodies are produced.

Fetus's red blood cells

Fetus's red blood cells destroyed

Woman's antibodies attacking fetus's red blood cells

Second Rh-positive fetus
Once an Rh-negative woman is Rh sensitized, the antibodies remain in her blood. If the woman becomes pregnant again and the fetus is Rh positive, the antibodies form in greater amounts. Destruction of a large number of the fetus's red blood cells causes anemia; because the red blood cells carry oxygen to the fetus, brain damage or even death may result.

CASE HISTORY
CONTROLLING DIABETES DURING PREGNANCY

MARILYN HAS HAD **diabetes (an abnormally high level of the sugar called glucose in the blood) since she was 16. She gives herself daily injections of insulin to bring the level of glucose down to normal. Marilyn knows diabetes can cause problems during pregnancy so, when she and her husband decided to start a family, she made an appointment to see her doctor.**

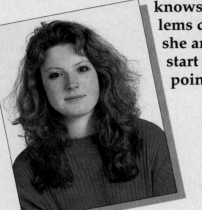

PERSONAL DETAILS
Name Marilyn Cooper
Age 24
Occupation Nurse
Family Both parents are well. Marilyn's sister and two brothers are also healthy.

MEDICAL BACKGROUND
Marilyn's diabetes is generally well controlled with insulin, although 2 years ago she had a severe attack of hypoglycemia (a low level of glucose in the blood).

THE CONSULTATION
Marilyn tells her doctor that she is not always careful about her diet and that her glucose levels, which she measures with a urine test, vary considerably. The doctor explains that diabetes increases the risk of having a baby with a birth defect, but that this risk can be greatly reduced if the level of glucose is carefully controlled before conception and throughout pregnancy.

Marilyn's doctor strongly encourages her to watch her diet more carefully in order to limit her intake of sugar. He also shows Marilyn how to test her blood glucose levels using a glucose meter, which provides more accurate results than the urine test, and how to adjust her dosage of insulin accordingly. He asks Marilyn to keep a daily record of her blood glucose levels and to come back to see him in 3 weeks.

THE DOCTOR'S EVALUATION
At her next appointment, Marilyn's records show that she now has WELL-CONTROLLED DIABETES and it is safe for her to try to become pregnant.

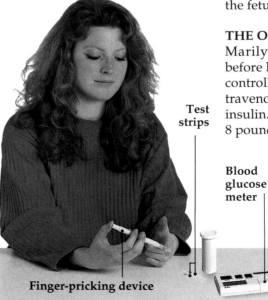

Test strips

Blood glucose meter

Finger-pricking device

PRENATAL CARE
Marilyn becomes pregnant 2 months later. She visits her obstetrician and her doctor frequently throughout her pregnancy. Her obstetrician examines her for signs of preeclampsia (high blood pressure brought on by pregnancy) and polyhydramnios (excess amniotic fluid). Her kidney function is also checked regularly. Marilyn's doctor tells her to monitor her blood glucose levels closely because her pregnancy will probably affect these levels. He tells her to call him immediately if she has severe vomiting or develops an infection; these may be signs that the dosage of her insulin must be changed.

Marilyn's pregnancy progresses well. She has weekly tests to check the fetus's heart rate and ultrasound scans to monitor its growth. The ultrasound scan at 33 weeks shows that the fetus is larger than normal, which is common among pregnant women with diabetes. Marilyn's doctor tells her that a large fetus, especially in a diabetic woman, can increase the risk of problems during delivery. He continues to monitor the fetus's growth very carefully.

THE OUTCOME
Marilyn's labor begins 10 days before her due date. Her diabetes is controlled during labor with an intravenous infusion of glucose and insulin. Marilyn delivers a healthy, 8 pound 8 ounce baby boy.

Testing her glucose level
Marilyn pricks her finger and applies a drop of blood to a test strip. She inserts the strip into a blood glucose meter, which reads the color of the strip and displays the glucose level. Marilyn needs more insulin during pregnancy to keep her glucose level down to normal.

MULTIPLE PREGNANCY

In a multiple pregnancy (meaning there is more than one fetus), both the woman and the fetuses are more likely to experience complications (see right). Multiple fetuses are at an increased risk of having a birth defect. Babies of multiple pregnancies are often born prematurely, are usually smaller, have lower birth weights, and have a higher rate of death during the first 2 weeks of life than single babies. Your doctor will monitor your diet to ensure that the fetuses' nutritional requirements are being met and may prescribe vitamin and mineral supplements (see page 61). After weeks 24 to 26 of pregnancy, some doctors recommend that the woman reduce her level of activity and have periodic ultrasound scans to monitor the growth of the fetuses.

MEDICAL CONDITIONS BEFORE PREGNANCY

If you have a medical condition, such as diabetes, see your doctor before you try to become pregnant. Some medical conditions increase the risk of complications during pregnancy.

High blood pressure

High blood pressure may interfere with the supply of oxygen and nutrients to the fetus, which can affect the growth of the fetus and require the baby to be delivered early. A pregnant woman with high blood pressure is more likely to have a heart attack or stroke or a stillbirth. If you have high blood pressure, your doctor will check carefully during pregnancy. He or she may prescribe blood pressure medication and perform tests to monitor the well-being of the fetus.

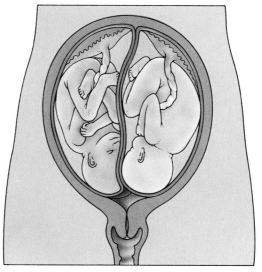

Risks of a multiple pregnancy
A woman with a multiple pregnancy is at increased risk of anemia, preeclampsia (high blood pressure brought on by pregnancy), or polyhydramnios (excess amniotic fluid), and of having an early and difficult labor.

Asthma

When carefully monitored and treated, asthma usually poses little risk during pregnancy to a woman or the fetus. In many women with mild asthma, the condition is often unaffected during pregnancy – and sometimes it even improves. However, severe asthma may worsen during pregnancy. Severe asthma attacks can reduce the oxygen supply to the fetus and may cause labor to start prematurely.

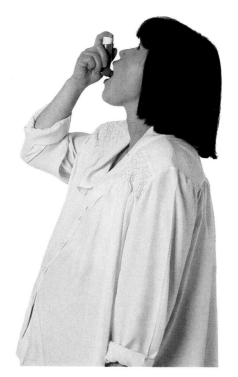

Asthma medications
As soon as you suspect you are pregnant, talk to your doctor about continuing to take asthma medication. Some asthma medications are considered safe for use during pregnancy. Any risk of taking these medications is minimal compared with the risk of harm to the fetus as a result of an asthma attack.

GESTATIONAL DIABETES

Some women develop a form of diabetes – a high level of glucose (a sugar) in the blood – during pregnancy. This condition, called gestational diabetes, usually goes away after the baby is born. A pregnant woman is at increased risk of developing gestational diabetes if she has close family members who have diabetes, has given birth previously to a baby who weighed more than 10 pounds, is seriously overweight, or has had a stillbirth for which the cause could not be determined. Your doctor may recommend that you have a glucose screening test (see page 56) to check for gestational diabetes.

URINARY TRACT INFECTION

About 10 percent of women develop at least one urinary tract infection during their pregnancy (see page 45). Prompt treatment with antibiotic drugs is important to clear up the infection and to avoid more serious complications that can affect both the woman and the fetus. If untreated, a urinary tract infection may bring on premature labor. Some doctors test a urine sample for a high level of bacteria at the first prenatal visit. A high level of bacteria may be present, yet not cause symptoms. The doctor may prescribe antibiotics to prevent the bacteria from causing a urinary tract infection.

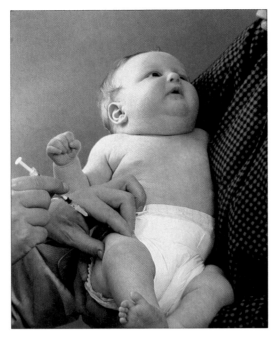

Preventing hepatitis B infection in a newborn
Hepatitis B infection of a newborn baby can be prevented by giving the baby an injection of antibodies shortly after birth, followed by a hepatitis B vaccine. A baby infected with the hepatitis B virus during delivery may become a carrier of the virus and is at risk of cirrhosis and cancer of the liver.

Liver disease

Hepatitis B is a viral infection that causes inflammation of the liver. Hepatitis B infection during pregnancy may result in premature labor and delivery. The hepatitis B virus can be passed to the baby during delivery if a woman has an active infection or is a carrier of the virus (which can remain in the body for years after the initial infection).

A pregnant woman with cirrhosis (a disease of the liver that impairs its function) is at risk of complications such as bleeding from the digestive tract and premature labor. The incidence of miscarriage and stillbirth is also increased in women with cirrhosis.

Heart disease

Heart disease is rare in women of childbearing age. About five to 10 out of 1,000 pregnant women are affected – usually as a result of damage to the heart caused by rheumatic fever or an abnormality that was present at birth. Because the heart must work harder during pregnancy, a woman with heart disease should consult her cardiologist (a heart specialist) before trying to conceive. Throughout pregnancy, monitoring by a cardiologist and an obstetrician is essential to help prevent complications.

Treatment for pregnant women with heart disease depends on the type and

TREATING EPILEPSY DURING PREGNANCY

A woman who has epilepsy should consult her doctor before becoming pregnant. A seizure that occurs during pregnancy can cause potentially life-threatening complications for both the woman and the fetus. Medications for epilepsy (called anticonvulsants) can increase the risk of fetal abnormalities.

Vitamin supplements
Anticonvulsant drugs reduce the absorption of folic acid and vitamin K into the bloodstream. Folic acid is essential for the formation of red blood cells in the woman and fetus and for the development of the fetus's nervous system, so many doctors prescribe folic acid supplements for a pregnant woman taking anticonvulsants. The baby is given an injection of vitamin K (essential for blood clotting) to prevent excessive bleeding as a result of a vitamin K deficiency.

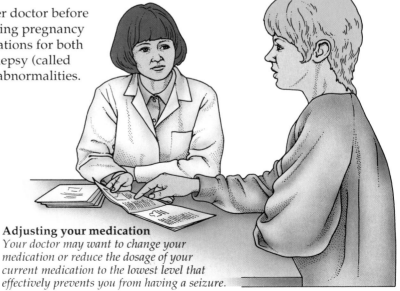

Adjusting your medication
Your doctor may want to change your medication or reduce the dosage of your current medication to the lowest level that effectively prevents you from having a seizure.

severity of the condition. Unless complications occur, most pregnant women who have heart disease are able to go into labor spontaneously at term and deliver the baby vaginally.

An overactive thyroid gland

Some women who have hyperthyroidism (an overactive thyroid gland) may be taking the drugs methimazole or propylthiouracil. Treatment with either of these drugs should continue during pregnancy. If an overactive thyroid gland is not controlled during pregnancy, this condition increases the risks of miscarriage, preeclampsia (high blood pressure brought on by pregnancy), premature labor, and infant death. Even with treatment, hyperthyroidism may worsen in the period just after childbirth.

Inherited blood disorders

Some inherited blood disorders, in which red blood cells contain abnormal types of hemoglobin (the oxygen-carrying part of these cells), can cause serious problems during pregnancy. The increased risks for a pregnant woman with sickle cell anemia are described at left. Another inherited blood disorder called thalassemia causes anemia as a result of the breakdown of blood cells. In a woman with thalassemia, the anemia is more likely to get worse during pregnancy.

Sickle cell anemia
In sickle cell anemia, some of the red blood cells become sickle-shaped (shown below, magnified 1,000 times). During pregnancy, sickle cell anemia increases the woman's risk of severe preeclampsia (high blood pressure brought on by pregnancy) and severe anemia. Blood vessels in the placenta can become blocked, leading to growth retardation or death of the fetus.

ASK YOUR DOCTOR
PROBLEMS DURING PREGNANCY

Q My wife has been treated for rheumatoid arthritis for the past 2 years. When she became pregnant 4 months ago, her doctor reduced her medication and she says she hasn't felt so well since before she got arthritis. What's going on?

A It is not unusual for a woman with rheumatoid arthritis or some other inflammatory disorders to feel better during pregnancy. Doctors think that increased hormone levels during pregnancy have an anti-inflammatory effect that temporarily relieves such conditions.

Q I take thyroxine for an underactive thyroid gland. Is this drug harmful during pregnancy?

A Thyroxine is not harmful to a fetus. Treatment with thyroxine should continue throughout pregnancy; a woman whose underactive thyroid gland is not treated during pregnancy has an increased risk of miscarriage.

Q I have systemic lupus erythematosus and just found out I am pregnant. Will this condition cause problems for me or my baby?

A Talk to your doctor as soon as possible. Systemic lupus erythematosus (a disorder of the tissues that hold structures of the body together) can increase the likelihood of blood clots and affect your kidney function. Your condition could also affect the development of the fetus's heart. Your doctor will counsel you about the risks of continuing the pregnancy. He or she may recommend prenatal tests and prescribe treatment to prevent problems.

MISCARRIAGE AND ECTOPIC PREGNANCY

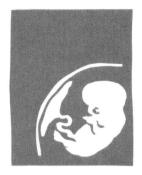

MOST PREGNANCIES progress naturally and normally and end with the uncomplicated delivery of a healthy baby. But sometimes the pregnancy ends prematurely and the fetus or embryo is lost – an event known as miscarriage. An ectopic pregnancy, in which the fertilized egg is implanted outside the uterus, also results in a premature end to a pregnancy.

Threatened miscarriage
In a threatened (possible) miscarriage, some blood is discharged from the vagina but the fetus remains alive in the uterus and the cervix remains closed. In about 50 percent of women who have a threatened miscarriage, the pregnancy continues normally to term.

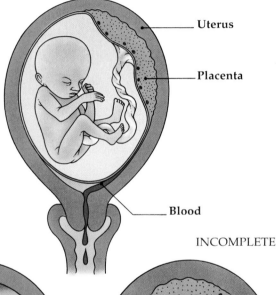

Uterus

Placenta

Blood

COMPLETE   INCOMPLETE

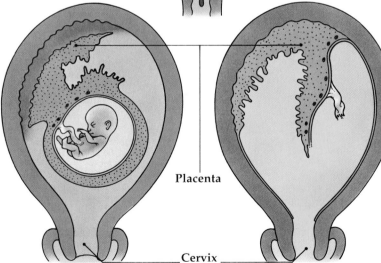

Placenta

Cervix

Impending miscarriage
In an impending (inevitable) miscarriage, the fetus has died and the cervix has dilated (widened). In a complete miscarriage, all of the fetal and placental tissue is expelled from the uterus (see above left). In an incomplete miscarriage, only some of the fetal or placental tissue is expelled (see above right). The tissue remaining in the uterus often causes bleeding and must be removed.

A miscarriage (or, in medical terminology, a spontaneous abortion) is the loss of the embryo or fetus before week 20 of a pregnancy, or before the fetus has developed sufficiently to survive outside the uterus. About 20 percent of all pregnancies end in a miscarriage, the majority occurring during the first trimester. The actual incidence of miscarriage is difficult to determine – some women miscarry before they know they are pregnant and mistake the vaginal bleeding for a late or heavy menstrual period, and not all women who have a miscarriage seek medical attention.

TYPES OF MISCARRIAGE

Any vaginal bleeding during the first trimester of pregnancy is considered a sign of a threatened (possible) miscarriage. A threatened miscarriage occurs in about one of five pregnant women. The bleeding may be accompanied by cramping pain in the lower part of the abdomen or by a low backache. You should be examined by your doctor immediately. He or she may recommend decreasing your level of activity or resting in bed until the bleeding stops.

An impending (inevitable) miscarriage occurs when the membrane of the amniotic sac has ruptured and the cervix has dilated (widened). In addition to the leakage of fluid, vaginal bleeding and abdominal cramping almost always occur. You should be examined by your doctor immediately. If the pregnancy is in the first trimester, you will be admitted to the hospital, where an operation called a dilation and curettage (D and C) will usually be done to remove the placental or fetal tissue. If the pregnancy is further along, your doctor may recommend that these tissues be allowed to empty from the uterus on their own; a D and C may be necessary.

A missed miscarriage occurs when the fetus has died during the early stages of the pregnancy but remains in the uterus. There may be slight vaginal bleeding or no bleeding at all. If your doctor suspects a missed miscarriage, an ultrasound scan may be done. If the diagnosis is confirmed, a D and C will be performed.

If a woman has miscarried three or more times, her doctor may recommend tests to determine the cause of the recurrent miscarriages. In such cases, the chances of carrying a future pregnancy to term depend on the factors that ended the previous pregnancies.

EMOTIONAL EFFECTS OF MISCARRIAGE

A miscarriage can have a profound effect on your emotions. A miscarriage should not be considered a sign that you will be unable to have a successful pregnancy. Early miscarriages are common and are, in fact, nature's selection process by which the body rejects an embryo because it is abnormal in some way. Some miscarriages are caused by health problems; usually these miscarriages cannot be prevented, but discuss any questions you have with your doctor.

The path to emotional recovery can be unsteady. Every woman needs time to grieve over her loss in her own way. Sometimes sharing these feelings of grief with your partner or a friend will help. You may want to ask your doctor for his or her recommendations for support groups or professional counseling.

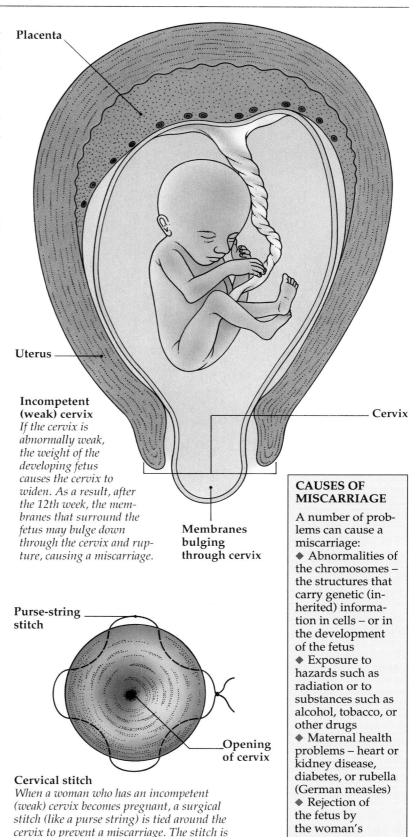

Placenta

Uterus

Incompetent (weak) cervix
If the cervix is abnormally weak, the weight of the developing fetus causes the cervix to widen. As a result, after the 12th week, the membranes that surround the fetus may bulge down through the cervix and rupture, causing a miscarriage.

Cervix

Membranes bulging through cervix

Purse-string stitch

Opening of cervix

Cervical stitch
When a woman who has an incompetent (weak) cervix becomes pregnant, a surgical stitch (like a purse string) is tied around the cervix to prevent a miscarriage. The stitch is usually removed at 37 weeks so that the woman can deliver the baby.

CAUSES OF MISCARRIAGE

A number of problems can cause a miscarriage:
◆ Abnormalities of the chromosomes – the structures that carry genetic (inherited) information in cells – or in the development of the fetus
◆ Exposure to hazards such as radiation or to substances such as alcohol, tobacco, or other drugs
◆ Maternal health problems – heart or kidney disease, diabetes, or rubella (German measles)
◆ Rejection of the fetus by the woman's immune system

ECTOPIC PREGNANCY

If a fertilized egg implants outside the uterus, it is called an ectopic pregnancy. About one in 100 pregnancies is ectopic. A woman who has had an ectopic pregnancy has a 10 to 20 percent chance of having another in a future pregnancy.

Most ectopic pregnancies occur in the fallopian tubes (see right). In many cases, the cause of an ectopic pregnancy cannot be determined, although some factors can increase the risk. For example, if a woman has had salpingitis (inflammation of the fallopian tubes), damage to tissues inside a tube may prevent an egg from passing through. Also, using an intrauterine device increases the chance of an ectopic pregnancy.

Symptoms of an ectopic pregnancy are lower abdominal pain (usually on one side), vaginal bleeding, and nausea and vomiting. These symptoms usually

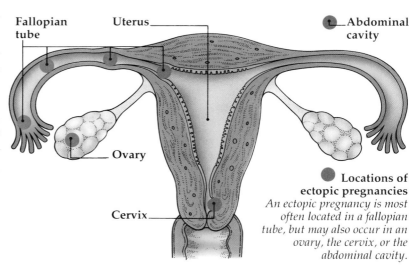

Locations of ectopic pregnancies
An ectopic pregnancy is most often located in a fallopian tube, but may also occur in an ovary, the cervix, or the abdominal cavity.

Ruptured ectopic pregnancy
Most ectopic pregnancies are diagnosed and terminated by 8 weeks. If a fertilized egg grows in the fallopian tube for longer than 10 weeks, its growth causes the tube to rupture. A ruptured ectopic pregnancy can cause life-threatening bleeding.

develop 6 weeks or more after the last menstrual period. If an ectopic pregnancy ruptures (see left), the abdominal pain becomes more severe as blood enters the abdominal cavity. The woman may experience pain in the shoulder and lightheadedness, and may even collapse.

Ectopic pregnancies often occur in women who are not aware that they are pregnant. If you have unexplainable abdominal pain, with or without vaginal bleeding, and there is a possibility that you could be pregnant, call your doctor immediately. Your doctor will examine you and order tests if he or she suspects an ectopic pregnancy. Blood tests, an ultrasound scan (see page 58), culdocentesis (insertion of a small needle through the vagina into the pelvic cavity to detect internal bleeding), and laparoscopy (see page 87) may be used to diagnose an ectopic pregnancy.

Treatment

A woman with a ruptured ectopic pregnancy needs immediate surgery to remove the embryo and any damaged tissue in the fallopian tube. In ectopic pregnancies that have not ruptured or are causing mild bleeding, the embryo can usually be removed surgically, using a laparoscope (see page 87). If possible, the fallopian tube is repaired; in some cases, it must be removed.

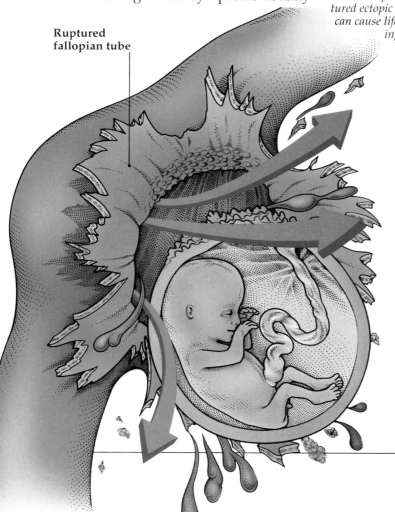

Ruptured fallopian tube

CASE HISTORY
A PAINFUL PREGNANCY

GINA AND HER HUSBAND TOM **had been trying to start a family and were thrilled when Gina's home pregnancy test indicated that she was pregnant. She immediately made an appointment to see her obstetrician.**

The next morning Gina woke up with a dull ache in her abdomen and noticed spots of blood on the bed sheets. Gina called her obstetrician, and he told her to come to his office right away.

PERSONAL DETAILS
Name Gina Viktora
Age 31
Occupation Realtor
Family Gina is an only child. Both her parents are healthy.

MEDICAL BACKGROUND
Three years ago Gina had salpingitis (inflammation of a fallopian tube) caused by an infection. Her obstetrician prescribed an antibiotic, and the condition cleared up.

THE CONSULTATION
Gina tells her obstetrician that she thinks she is pregnant and is very worried about her abdominal pain and bleeding. The obstetrician asks Gina to provide a urine sample for another pregnancy test, which is again positive. He examines Gina's abdomen and performs an internal (pelvic) examination. He finds a tender area above Gina's pubic bone and a lump in the lower right side of her abdomen. He arranges for Gina to have an ultrasound scan at the hospital immediately.

THE DIAGNOSIS
AND TREATMENT
The ultrasound scan does not show a fetus in Gina's uterus and indicates that her right fallopian tube is much thicker than normal. The obstetrician tells Gina that he suspects an ECTOPIC PREGNANCY. He explains to her that salpingitis may have damaged a fallopian tube and caused the fertilized egg to implant in the tube instead of the uterus. He recommends that Gina be operated on immediately because the growing embryo will cause the fallopian tube to rupture. Gina agrees and is taken to the operating room.

With the use of a laparoscope (see below), the diagnosis is confirmed and the embryo and damaged tissue from the fallopian tube are removed. Gina recovers well and is released from the hospital the next day.

THE OUTCOME
Gina sees her obstetrician several days later. She tells him she is worried she will never have a successful pregnancy. Her doctor explains that the damage to her fallopian tube should heal and chances are good that she will be able to become pregnant again, although there is some risk of another ectopic pregnancy. He advises Gina to come see him early in her next pregnancy. Eight months later, Gina suspects she is pregnant and goes to see her obstetrician immediately. She is delighted when he confirms she is 8 weeks pregnant and everything is normal.

Laparoscopic investigation and surgery
Gina's ectopic pregnancy is confirmed using a viewing instrument called a laparoscope that is inserted through a small incision. The embryo and damaged tissue from the fallopian tube are also removed through the laparoscope.

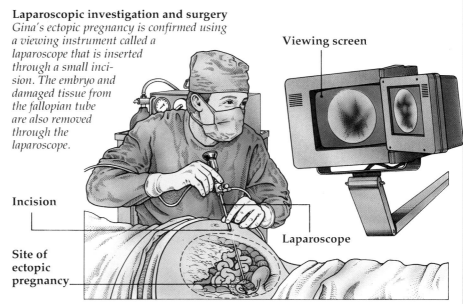

Viewing screen

Incision

Laparoscope

Site of ectopic pregnancy

CHAPTER FOUR

LABOR AND DELIVERY

WOMEN'S ATTITUDES toward and expectations about labor and delivery have changed tremendously over the years. Although childbirth was once a dreaded occurrence, most women now view it as a positive experience and want to learn as much as they can about what to expect at this important time. In the past, labor was often a painful and frightening event that sometimes lasted many days. Babies were born at home, often without the assistance of a medical professional. The risk to the woman's health and her life was considerable. Bleeding and infection were common causes of death among women who gave birth. Many babies died during labor or in the first week of life, and many others were born physically or mentally handicapped as a result of injury during birth. Most women today are well prepared for

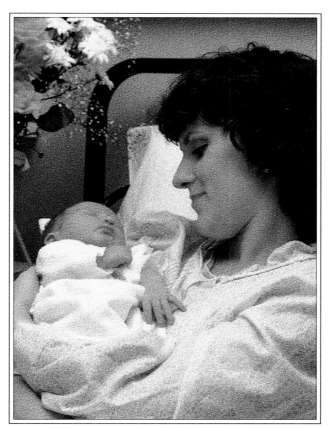

labor and childbirth. Most babies are now born in a hospital after a labor that has been carefully monitored. Medical advances such as the use of antibiotic drugs, sophisticated electronic monitoring equipment, and improved surgical and anesthetic techniques have helped to substantially reduce the numbers of deaths of both mother and child. Although practices such as giving an enema, shaving of the pubic area, an episiotomy, using stirrups, or giving drugs for pain relief may be necessary during childbirth, they can sometimes be matters of choice for the woman. Many women now have their partners or family members present throughout labor and at the birth to provide comfort, support, and assistance. In this chapter, we explain several forms of intervention that may be necessary during the birth of your baby. In some cases, problems develop that make it impossible or dangerous to deliver a baby vaginally. In such cases, the doctor will deliver the baby by cesarean section. The advent of epidural anesthesia has enabled women to be conscious during a cesarean so that they can witness the baby's birth. Complications occasionally occur during or after childbirth. For example, vaginal tissue may be torn during the birth and may need to be stitched. The sight of your newborn baby will be a source of wonder for you and your partner and you will want to examine every detail of his or her appearance and behavior to reassure yourselves that everything is normal. Once your baby has arrived and you are adjusting to the new challenges of caring for your baby, you should not forget to take care of yourself as your body recovers from the changes and demands of pregnancy and childbirth.

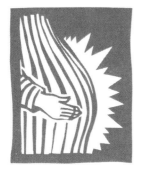

HOW LABOR BEGINS

NEW CHANGES OCCUR in your body during the last weeks of pregnancy that are signs of the approaching birth. Just as each woman's pregnancy progresses differently, the start of labor is also a unique process. Childbirth rarely occurs without plenty of warning signs that labor is beginning. Recognizing and understanding these signs will help ease any fears you may have and better prepare you for the process of labor.

ARE YOU READY?

As your delivery date draws closer, make a list of important phone numbers – your partner, family, babysitter, and taxicab, as well as your doctor and the hospital – and keep it handy. Make a couple of trial runs at different times of day so you know how long it takes to get to the hospital.

The exact mechanism in a woman's body that triggers the beginning of labor is not known. Some researchers propose that an interaction of hormones between the woman and fetus initiates labor.

SIGNS OF LABOR

Some changes in your body are early signs that labor is approaching. You may lose a few pounds near the time of your due date. You may also feel more com-fortable and notice that your clothes fit differently – a sign that the fetus has "dropped" down into the bony part of your pelvis (called engagement – see below). The following signs indicate that labor is imminent; you should call your doctor as soon as possible.

A plug of mucus

As the fetus pushes against the cervix, the cervix begins to widen and the plug of mucus that has sealed off the uterus

Engagement
When the fetus moves down in the woman's abdomen ("drops") and settles into the pelvis, this is called engagement. Engagement usually occurs 2 to 4 weeks before labor. In a woman who has already had a baby, engage-ment may not occur until labor begins.

NOT
ENGAGED

ENGAGED

Pelvis

comes loose. When this plug of mucus, mixed with a small amount of blood, is expelled, it is called the "show." Labor usually begins within a few days.

Your water breaks

A gush or trickle of fluid from the vagina is a sign that the membranes of the amniotic sac (called the "bag of waters") has broken. The bag of waters may break before labor starts or during the first stage of labor. The amniotic fluid is usually clear. If the fluid looks dark (green, brown, or yellow) or smells unpleasant, the fetus probably had a bowel movement, which may indicate that the fetus was or is stressed (see page 97). If contractions have not started within 12 to 24 hours after your water breaks, your doctor may decide to induce labor because there is a risk of infection. Labor may be induced earlier if the fetus shows signs of being stressed.

Strong contractions

During the last 3 months of pregnancy you may experience erratic, light, usually painless contractions called Braxton Hicks contractions. This type of contraction does not signal the start of labor, but rather helps stretch the muscles of the uterus in preparation for labor. Contractions that become progressively stronger and occur at regular intervals are a sign of labor. Some women experience labor contractions as pain in the lower part of the abdomen accompanied by a hardening of the abdominal wall. Other women feel an aching across the lower part of the back. Time your contractions by counting from the beginning of one contraction to the beginning of the next. Initially, the contractions are infrequent – sometimes 20 to 30 minutes apart. When the contractions are occurring regularly, at least once every 2 to 10 minutes, labor has usually started. The intensity, frequency, and duration of the contractions will increase as the time for the birth of your baby approaches.

CHANGES IN THE CERVIX

The cervix is the thick, firm band of muscles at the lower part of the uterus. The cervix undergoes changes during the late stages of pregnancy and during labor in preparation for delivery of the baby.

1 The cervix gradually softens as a result of hormone changes.

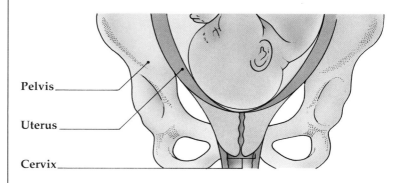

Pelvis

Uterus

Cervix

2 Contractions of the muscles of the uterus then gently pull the cervix upward, making it longer and thinner.

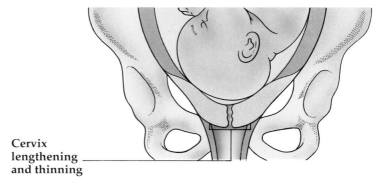

Cervix lengthening and thinning

3 The contractions cause the opening of the cervix to gradually dilate (widen). The membranes of the amniotic sac (the "bag of waters") may break at this stage.

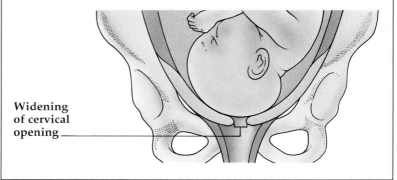

Widening of cervical opening

MONITOR YOUR SYMPTOMS
AM I IN LABOR?

The average length of pregnancy is 40 weeks, but it is quite normal for a baby to be born any time between 37 and 42 weeks. A number of different signs – abdominal or back pains, the passage of a plug of mucus, and rupture of the amniotic sac (the "bag of waters") – are indications that labor may begin soon. The signs of labor experienced by each woman and the order in which they occur vary. This chart is designed to help you recognize when labor has started.

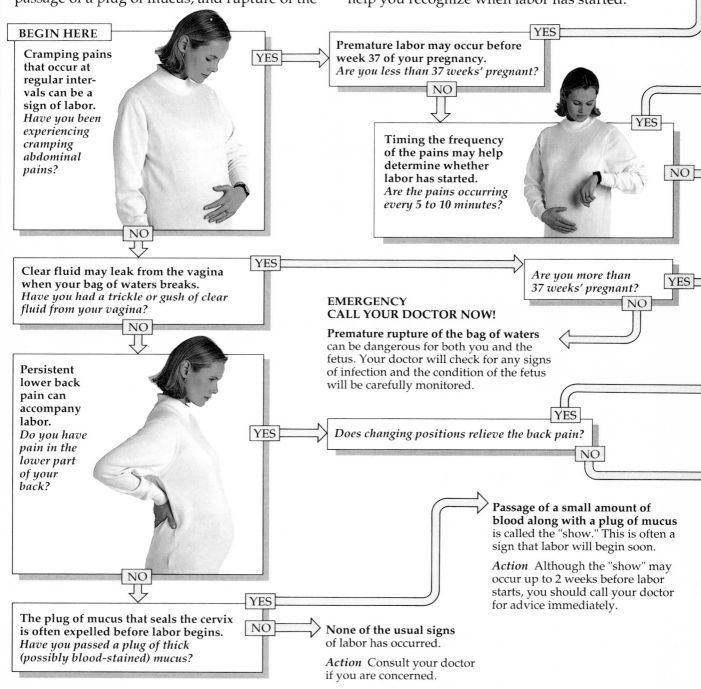

BEGIN HERE

Cramping pains that occur at regular intervals can be a sign of labor.
Have you been experiencing cramping abdominal pains?

YES

Premature labor may occur before week 37 of your pregnancy.
Are you less than 37 weeks' pregnant?

YES

NO

Timing the frequency of the pains may help determine whether labor has started.
Are the pains occurring every 5 to 10 minutes?

YES

NO

NO

Clear fluid may leak from the vagina when your bag of waters breaks.
Have you had a trickle or gush of clear fluid from your vagina?

YES

Are you more than 37 weeks' pregnant?

YES

NO

NO

**EMERGENCY
CALL YOUR DOCTOR NOW!**

Premature rupture of the bag of waters can be dangerous for both you and the fetus. Your doctor will check for any signs of infection and the condition of the fetus will be carefully monitored.

Persistent lower back pain can accompany labor.
Do you have pain in the lower part of your back?

YES

Does changing positions relieve the back pain?

YES

NO

Passage of a small amount of blood along with a plug of mucus is called the "show." This is often a sign that labor will begin soon.

Action Although the "show" may occur up to 2 weeks before labor starts, you should call your doctor for advice immediately.

NO

The plug of mucus that seals the cervix is often expelled before labor begins.
Have you passed a plug of thick (possibly blood-stained) mucus?

YES

NO

None of the usual signs of labor has occurred.

Action Consult your doctor if you are concerned.

EMERGENCY CALL YOUR DOCTOR NOW!

Premature labor may be stopped if you seek immediate medical attention.

CALL YOUR DOCTOR NOW!

Regular contractions of the muscles of the uterus are a sign that labor is starting. Leakage of fluid from your vagina and the passage of a plug of mucus may also occur.

Action Call your doctor. He or she will tell you what to do next.

The early stages of labor may be signaled by occasional cramping pains in the abdomen. These pains are caused by contraction of the muscles of the uterus. The contractions will become stronger and more frequent as labor progresses.

Action Time your contractions and call your doctor. When contractions occur regularly every 10 minutes, labor has probably started. Call your doctor immediately if you have any leakage of fluid from the vagina.

Rupture of the bag of waters sometimes occurs several hours before contractions start, although the bag of waters usually breaks during the early stages of labor.

Action Contact your doctor immediately if your bag of waters breaks. He or she may tell you to go to the hospital or advise you to wait at home until contractions begin. If contractions do not start on their own, your doctor may induce labor.

Pain in the lower part of your back that is relieved by changing your position is usually not a sign that labor has started.

Action To help relieve back pain, try lying on your side or sitting in a semireclining position with a pillow under your knees. Call your doctor for advice if you are more than 37 weeks pregnant and the back pain has lasted for more than an hour, or if you have any vaginal bleeding and/or have passed a plug of mucus.

Persistent back pain that occurs during the last few weeks of pregnancy can be a sign of labor. Cramping abdominal pain may develop several hours after the back pain started. Back pain may, however, be a sign of a kidney infection.

Action Call your doctor for advice.

WHAT TO BRING TO THE HOSPITAL

About 2 weeks before your delivery date, you should pack a bag with the personal things – for you and your baby – that you want to take to the hospital. Below is a list of items you may want to include. And don't forget to have someone bring a car seat for the baby for the trip home.

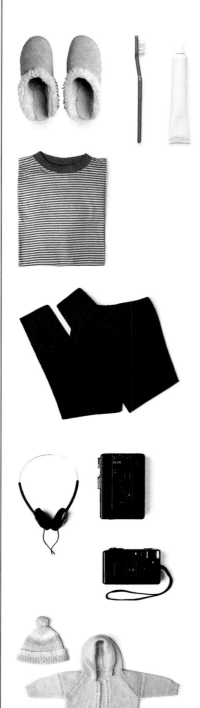

FOR YOU
◆ Nightgown (opening in the front if you plan to breast-feed)
◆ Robe
◆ Thick socks
◆ Slippers
◆ Underpants
◆ Bras (nursing bras if you plan to breast-feed)
◆ Clothes to wear home
◆ Toothbrush and toothpaste
◆ Deodorant
◆ Moisturizing lotion
◆ Lip balm or small jar of petroleum jelly
◆ Brush and comb
◆ Elastic bands or barrettes to hold back your hair
◆ Shampoo and conditioner
◆ Hand-held hair dryer (can be used to dry stitches so as to avoid rubbing sensitive areas)
◆ Bag to hold dirty laundry
◆ Breast pads (to absorb leaking milk)
◆ Eyeglasses
◆ Books or magazines
◆ Camera, flash, and batteries
◆ Portable stereo with headphones and tapes
◆ Telephone numbers of friends and relatives

FOR YOUR BABY
◆ Undershirt
◆ Sleeper
◆ Blanket
◆ Sweater and hat

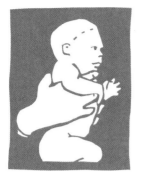

THE STAGES OF LABOR

LABOR OCCURS in three stages. In the first stage, the woman experiences contractions of the muscles of the uterus that cause the cervix to dilate (widen) so that the baby can pass down into the vagina. During the second stage, aided by the woman's pushing, the baby passes through the vagina and is delivered. In the third stage, the placenta is expelled from the uterus.

Dilation of the cervix
During labor for a first baby, the cervical opening dilates (widens) about 1 centimeter (about ½ inch) per hour. The cervix may dilate more rapidly in a woman who has already had a baby. When the cervix is fully dilated (10 centimeters – just under 4 inches), the baby's head begins to press through the cervix toward the vagina.

Just as every woman's pregnancy is unique, so is childbirth. In most women, labor lasts an average of 12 to 14 hours for a first baby. Subsequent labors are shorter, usually lasting about 7 hours.

FIRST STAGE

The first stage of labor is usually the longest – about 8 to 10 hours. Contractions of the muscles of the uterus cause the cervix to dilate (see below). In the early phase, the contractions may be mild and infrequent. Contractions then gradually become stronger and more regular. During the active phase of the first stage of labor, contractions usually occur 3 to 4 minutes apart. Once contractions are 2 to 3 minutes apart, the cervix is usually almost fully dilated.

Most women spend the early phase of labor at home. Once the contractions become stronger and more frequent, you should start timing the contractions and call your doctor. He or she will tell you when to leave for the hospital.

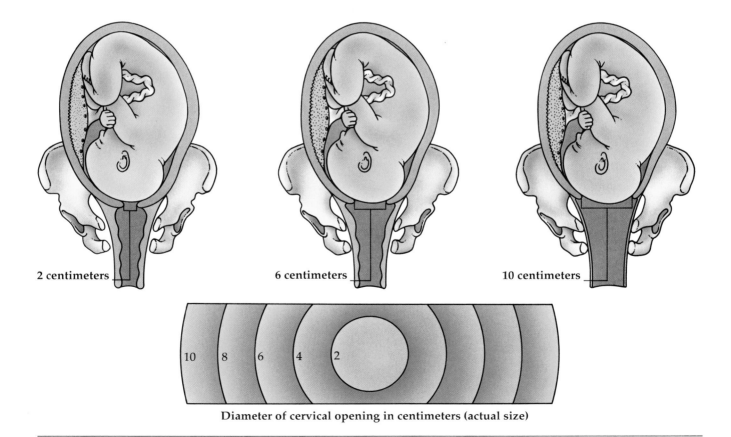

2 centimeters   6 centimeters   10 centimeters

Diameter of cervical opening in centimeters (actual size)

COMFORTABLE POSITIONS DURING THE FIRST STAGE OF LABOR

During the first stage of labor, the most important thing you can do is to try to relax. Relaxation can help decrease the discomfort of labor, helps conserve your energy, and allows the contractions to be more efficient because the uterus is not constricted by tightened abdominal muscles. Many women feel most relaxed and comfortable walking around during the first stage of labor. Others find the positions described below to be more comfortable.

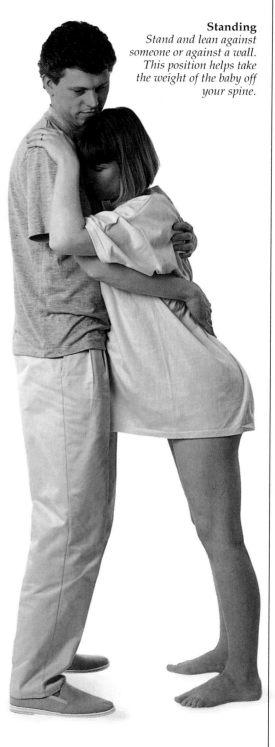

Standing
Stand and lean against someone or against a wall. This position helps take the weight of the baby off your spine.

On your hands and knees
Get down on your hands and knees and gently rock backward and forward during contractions. Do not arch your back. Between contractions, fold your arms and lean forward, resting your head on your arms.

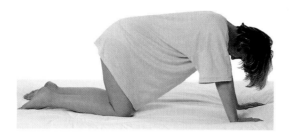

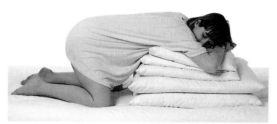

Kneeling forward
Kneel on the floor or a bed, with your knees comfortably apart, and lean forward onto a stack of pillows.

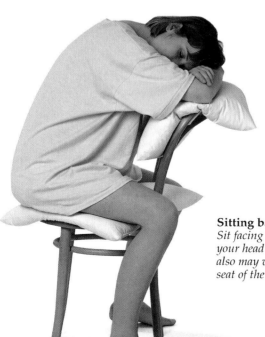

Sitting backward
Sit facing the back of a chair and rest your head and arms on a pillow. You also may want to put a pillow on the seat of the chair.

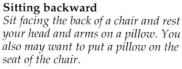

HOW PAIN MEDICATIONS ARE GIVEN DURING LABOR AND DELIVERY

During your prenatal visits with your doctor, you should discuss what type of pain medication (if any) you want during labor and delivery (see page 51). Some women prefer not to receive any pain medication. However, there are times when pain medication may be necessary – such as when labor is very long or complicated, if the pain becomes more than the woman is able to tolerate or interferes with her ability to push, in breech deliveries (see page 104), or when forceps must be used (see page 109).

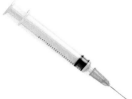

Intravenous and intramuscular injections

A variety of painkillers can be given intravenously (injected directly into a vein or by an intravenous drip) or intramuscularly (injected into a muscle, usually in the buttocks). Painkillers given in this way take effect quickly and pain relief lasts up to 2 hours. However, these painkillers can sometimes cause side effects such as nausea, vomiting, dizziness, and confusion. Your doctor will carefully time the administration of these drugs during labor so that they will not adversely affect the baby; if given just before delivery, the baby's ability to breathe can be impaired.

How is epidural anesthesia given?

An infusion of fluids by intravenous drip is started. A hollow needle is then inserted into the epidural space (the space between the bones of the spine and the membrane covering the spinal cord) while you are lying down with your knees up and your back rounded or while you are sitting with your back rounded. A soft tube (called a catheter), attached to a syringe, is passed through the needle, and an anesthetic (which numbs the nerves that supply the lower part of the abdomen, the pelvis, and sometimes the legs) is injected. The needle is removed, and the part of the tube that protrudes from your back is taped down. You do not feel the tube, which allows more anesthetic to be given if needed. Possible side effects are slowing of contractions, reduced ability to push, and inability to empty the bladder if necessary during labor. A catheter may be inserted into the bladder to empty it periodically.

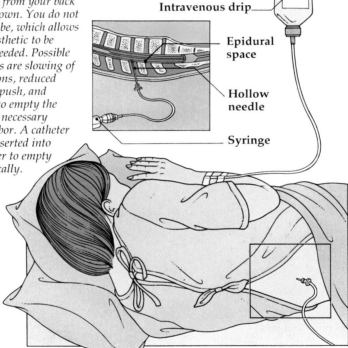

Intravenous drip

Epidural space

Hollow needle

Syringe

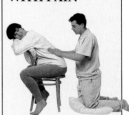

COPING WITH PAIN

Instead of relying on medication to relieve pain, prepared (or natural) childbirth uses techniques for breathing and relaxation (such as massage and mental imagery) – taught to both the expectant mother and her partner – to help the woman cope with pain during labor and delivery. The support and reassurance given by her partner help reduce any fears and, as a result, help the woman to better tolerate pain.

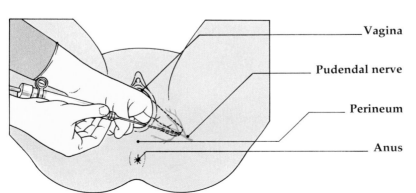

Vagina

Pudendal nerve

Perineum

Anus

Pudendal block

A pudendal block is injection of an anesthetic (such as lidocaine) into the tissues surrounding the pudendal nerves, one on each side of the vagina (see left). The medication blocks pain in the vaginal and perineal area (the tissues between the vaginal opening and the anus). A pudendal block is given for pain relief during the delivery of the baby; it does not relieve the pain of labor. This type of anesthetic takes effect quickly and has no serious side effects.

FETAL MONITORING

Labor can be stressful for your baby as well as for you. A technique called electronic fetal monitoring is sometimes used (either continuously or at various times throughout labor and delivery) to provide information on how well the baby is tolerating the stress of labor. This technique monitors the response of the baby's heart to the contractions of the uterus and alerts the doctor to any signs that the baby is having trouble so that immediate action can be taken.

How is monitoring done?

Monitoring can be done externally or internally. External fetal monitoring uses two electronic devices placed on the woman's abdomen (see below). The baby's heart rate can also be checked externally with a special stethoscope. If done at properly timed intervals, this type of monitoring is as effective as electronic monitoring.

If a more accurate measurement is required (such as when the baby is having trouble), the baby's heart rate may be recorded by an electrode passed through the vagina and placed on the baby's scalp; this is internal fetal monitoring. With an internal monitor on the baby (see page 113), contractions can be measured by a device on the woman's abdomen or by a tube inserted into the uterus.

The changing heartbeat

A change in the baby's normal heartbeat pattern is often the first sign of stress. If the baby becomes more stressed, his or her heart rate tends to consistently slow after a contraction and takes longer to return to normal. If the baby is severely stressed, the heart rate may drop below 100 beats per minute or may increase above 160 beats per minute.

SIGN OF STRESS

Inside the uterus, a baby's intestines are filled with a mixture of amniotic fluid that the baby has swallowed and mucus from the bowel. This mixture is called meconium. If a baby becomes stressed, even temporarily, its intestines can contract and force meconium out of the baby's anus into the amniotic fluid. If your amniotic fluid is stained (green or brown) with meconium it may indicate your baby is stressed, and your doctor may monitor your labor closely.

EXTERNAL FETAL MONITORING

In external fetal monitoring, two devices are placed on the woman's abdomen. One (an ultrasound transducer) picks up the baby's heartbeat. The other is a pressure-sensitive gauge that measures the frequency and duration of the woman's contractions. A monitor shows and prints out the readings.

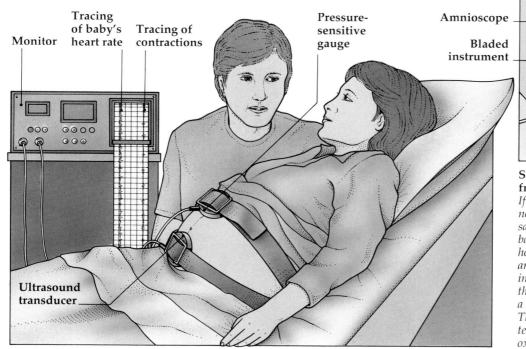

Monitor — Tracing of baby's heart rate — Tracing of contractions — Pressure-sensitive gauge — Ultrasound transducer

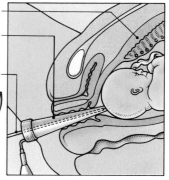

Uterus — Amnioscope — Bladed instrument

Sampling blood from the baby's scalp
If your baby's heart rate is abnormal, your doctor may take a sample of blood through the baby's scalp. The doctor puts a hollow instrument called an amnioscope into the uterus, then inserts a bladed instrument through the amnioscope to make a tiny slit in the baby's scalp. The blood sample is tested to determine if the baby has enough oxygen in its bloodstream.

SECOND STAGE

The second stage of labor begins when you start to push your baby out of the uterus and into the vagina and ends when your baby is born. This stage usually takes 40 to 60 minutes for a first baby and 15 to 30 minutes for a second baby. Once the cervix is fully dilated, your doctor will tell you to start pushing during the contractions. Pushing before the cervix is fully dilated can cause the tissues of the cervix to swell or tear. Aided by the woman's pushing and the contractions of the uterus, the baby's head is pushed down through the pelvis. Usually the baby first enters the pelvis with his or her head facing sideways and then rotates around to face downward.

Pushing positions

Various positions can be used for the pushing stage of labor. Some hospitals and doctors prefer certain positions so you should discuss this subject with your doctor during your prenatal visits. You may find sitting with your knees apart in a semireclining position in bed to be the most comfortable position (see below). Or you may prefer to be on your

THE BIRTH OF YOUR BABY

1 When delivery is about to occur, your baby's head will expand the vaginal opening, causing the anus and the perineum (the area between the vaginal opening and the anus) to bulge. The doctor will ask you to push with each contraction.

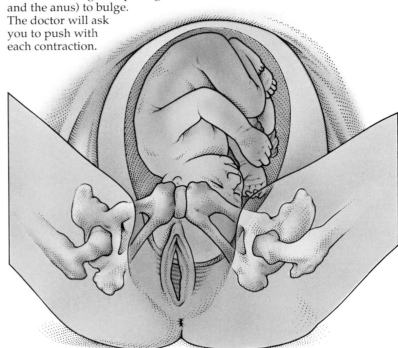

2 As your baby's head emerges, your doctor will ask you to take quick breaths and not to push. This allows the doctor to control the delivery of your baby's head, letting the vaginal tissues stretch gently and reducing the likelihood that the tissues of the perineum will tear.

Pushing in a semireclining position
At the start of a contraction, sit with your knees apart and hold the outside of your thighs. Draw your legs toward you and take a deep breath. Tuck your chin into your chest, hold your breath, and push downward. Push for a count of 10 seconds, then exhale, take another deep breath, and repeat this pattern until the contraction is over. Rest between the contractions by relaxing your muscles and breathing evenly.

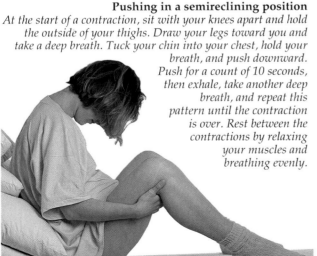

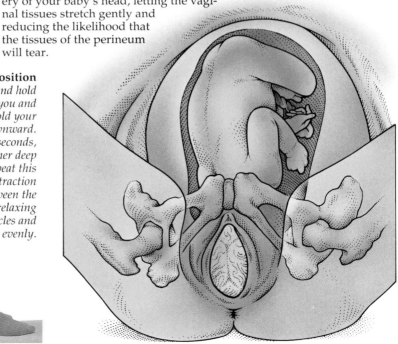

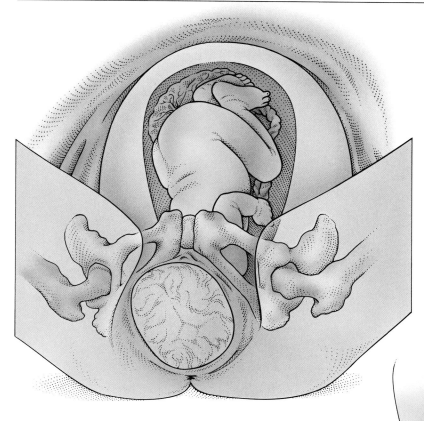

3 Usually your baby's head will be facing downward toward the anus, and then your baby will turn sideways as his or her shoulders enter your pelvis.

4 The doctor will clear any fluid from your baby's nose and mouth and check to see if the umbilical cord is wrapped around his or her neck. If it is, the cord will be gently lifted over your baby's head or will be clamped and cut. The next contraction is usually enough to make the shoulders emerge. Your baby then slides out.

5 The umbilical cord is clamped in two places and is cut between the clamps. Cutting the umbilical cord does not hurt your baby.

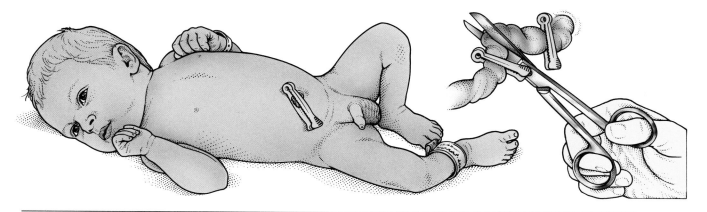

hands and knees, to squat on a bed (facing your partner, with your arms around your partner's neck or shoulders) or on the floor (usually supported from behind by your partner), or to use a birthing stool (somewhat like sitting on a toilet).

THIRD STAGE

The third stage of labor lasts from the birth of the baby until the delivery of the placenta (called the afterbirth) – usually about 5 to 15 minutes. After the baby is born, the uterus continues to contract, although the contractions are less painful. The placenta separates from the wall of the uterus and moves into the lower part of the uterus or into the vagina. The woman may be able to push the placenta out or the doctor may help remove it (see right). The doctor then carefully examines the placenta and the membranes that surrounded the baby to make sure all the tissue has been expelled.

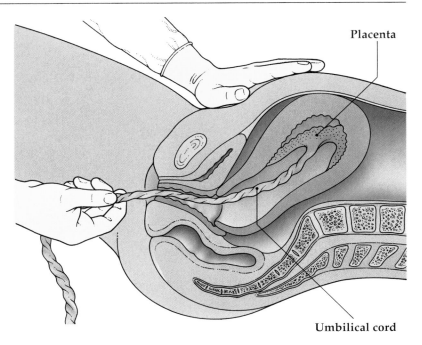

Placenta

Umbilical cord

Delivering the placenta
To help deliver the placenta, the doctor may put one hand on your abdomen and gently pull on the umbilical cord with his or her other hand as you push the placenta out.

FIRST MOMENTS WITH YOUR BABY

After the umbilical cord has been cut and your baby's condition has been evaluated, he or she will be given to you to hold. If there is any cause for concern about your baby's breathing, a pediatrician will treat that first. You may choose to breast-feed your baby right away. Breast-feeding sometimes strengthens your contractions, which helps in the delivery of the placenta.

Holding your baby
After his or her bath, your baby is dressed in a diaper and gown, wrapped in a blanket, and given back to you to hold.

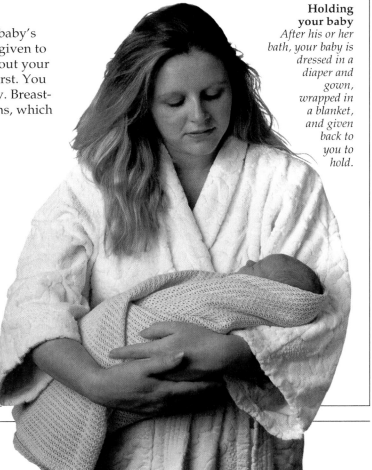

Baby's first bath
After you have held your new baby for the first time, a nurse will bathe him or her. The bathing is usually done in the delivery room.

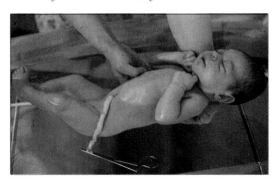

DELIVERING TWINS

Twins must be closely monitored throughout labor to ensure that the placenta is supplying both babies with oxygen. Initially, external fetal monitoring (see page 97) is used for both babies; after the amniotic sac ruptures (the "bag of waters" breaks), an electrode is often applied to the scalp of the twin who will be delivered first.

After the first baby has been delivered, the doctor determines the position of the second baby. If the second baby is lying head down and its heartbeat is normal, labor may proceed on its own. If the second baby is lying horizontally, the doctor may be able to turn the baby to a head-down or a breech position (see EX-TERNAL VERSION on page 73). If the baby cannot be turned, it must be delivered by cesarean section.

Bleeding is more common after delivery of twins than after delivery of one baby because the site at which the placenta was attached to the wall of the uterus is larger and the number of blood vessels affected is greater. Also, the uterus has stretched more and may not contract as well, resulting in bleeding. After both babies are born, the doctor may give the woman an injection of oxytocin (see page 107) to help the uterus contract and prevent excessive bleeding.

Delivery of twins
After the doctor has delivered the first baby, he or she clamps the first baby's umbilical cord to prevent any risk of the second baby bleeding from this cord. Such bleeding can occur with identical twins (who develop from one egg) because the babies share the same placenta.

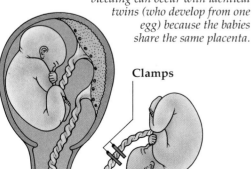

Clamps

Twin positions
In most cases the head or buttocks of one or both twins face downward, but occasionally one or both babies lie horizontally. An ultrasound scan may be done late in your pregnancy to determine the positions of the twins. Some possible combinations are shown below; the frequency of each combination is in parentheses.

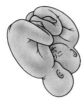

Both twins head down (45 percent)

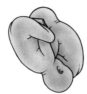

Head down and buttocks down (37 percent)

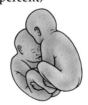

Both twins buttocks down (10 percent)

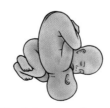

Head down and horizontal (5 percent)

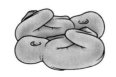

Both twins horizontal (1/2 percent)

ASK YOUR DOCTOR CHILDBIRTH

Q My doctor told me he uses fetal monitoring for all births. A friend told me that if a fetal monitor is used I may be more likely to have a cesarean. Is this true?

A You should talk to your doctor about the circumstances for which he or she recommends a cesarean section. The connection between fetal monitoring and the rate of cesarean sections is controversial. In some cases, fetal monitoring may have resulted in a high rate of detection of potentially life-threatening problems of the fetus for which a cesarean section is recommended.

Q When I visited the hospital where I will soon be delivering my baby, I saw a woman being taken from the delivery room with an intravenous drip. Is this routine?

A Many doctors give a solution of nutrients and fluid intravenously during labor. This practice ensures that you don't become dehydrated and provides a means of giving medication if needed. Talk to your doctor about the circumstances for which he or she feels intravenous fluids might be necessary.

Q I am worried that I may embarrass myself by having a bowel movement when I push during labor. I don't want to have an enema, but what else can I do?

A When labor begins, most women need to use the bathroom frequently and have loose bowel movements that often empty the colon. If you do have a bowel movement while pushing, be reassured that the staff has seen this many times and will clean up immediately.

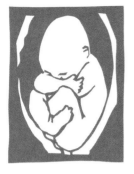

PROBLEMS OF LABOR

IT IS REASSURING to remember that most labors and deliveries proceed without complications. However, problems can occur. Weak or inefficient contractions can slow or stop the progress of labor. Sometimes, because of the baby's size or position, his or her passage through the woman's pelvis is difficult or impossible.

During labor, the contractions of the uterus normally follow a well-coordinated pattern and start in the upper part of the uterus (see below). If the pattern of the contractions is not coordinated or if the contractions are too weak to be effective, the progress of labor is altered.

INEFFECTIVE CONTRACTIONS

During labor, contractions sometimes start in the middle of the uterus and spread in a random pattern. These contractions are just as frequent and painful as coordinated contractions but may not cause the cervix to dilate (widen). The progress of labor will be slow. If the contractions remain abnormal, a cesarean section may need to be performed before the baby becomes stressed.

Contractions that are too weak can sometimes be strengthened by rupturing the membranes of the amniotic sac (see page 107). Weak contractions can also be strengthened by giving the woman the drug oxytocin, a hormone that stimulates contractions (see page 107). Sometimes during labor, contractions begin normally and then stop

Contractions of the uterus
During labor, the upper part of the uterus normally contracts more strongly than the lower part (see right) and the baby is pushed downward and out through the birth canal (the passage extending from the cervix to the vaginal opening). Sometimes, the pattern of the contractions is reversed, with the strongest contractions occurring in the lower part of the uterus, and the baby cannot be pushed down into the birth canal (see far right). The doctor may give the woman the drug oxytocin to increase the effectiveness of the contractions. If this treatment is not successful, a cesarean section is necessary.

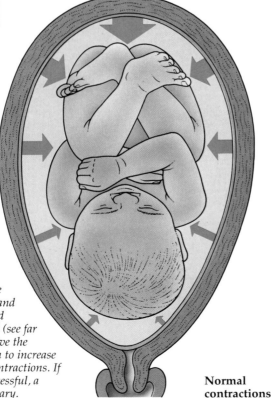

Normal contractions

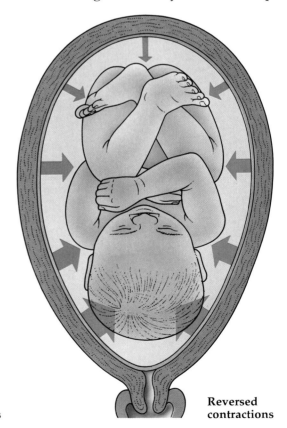

Reversed contractions

suddenly. Before giving oxytocin to try to start the contractions again, the doctor checks to make sure the baby is lying in the proper position and that there is no deformity of the woman's pelvis or other factors that may be obstructing the passage of the baby.

THE BIRTH CANAL

Sometimes, despite strong contractions of the uterus, the cervix does not dilate. This problem may be caused by fibrosis (scar tissue) if the woman has had extensive surgery on the cervix or may be caused by fibroids (noncancerous tumors) in the cervix. A cesarean section may be required to deliver the baby.

Fibroids in the uterus
Fibroids (noncancerous tumors) in the wall of the uterus may prevent the uterus from contracting normally or may block the passage of the baby. The baby may need to be delivered by cesarean section.

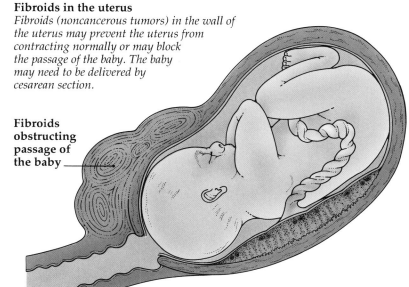

Fibroids obstructing passage of the baby

ROUND PELVIS

Pelvic inlet
13 centimeters
(average diameter)

Pelvic outlet
11 centimeters
(average diameter)

HEART-SHAPED PELVIS

Pelvic inlet
12 centimeters
(average diameter)

Pelvic outlet
10 centimeters
(average diameter)

Pelvic shape and size

Pelvic abnormalities can stop the baby from passing into the birth canal (the passage extending from the cervix to the vaginal opening). Osteomalacia (weakening of bones caused by a vitamin D deficiency) can cause abnormalities in the size and shape of a woman's pelvis. A previous fracture of a pelvic bone can change the shape of a woman's pelvis.

The size of the woman's pelvis in relation to the size of the baby's head is a crucial factor that influences the ease of labor and delivery. If the woman's pelvis is too small to allow the baby to pass through (either because of the structure of the pelvic bones or because the baby is very large), the baby cannot drop down far enough for the head to become engaged at the entrance to the birth canal (see page 90). In such a case, a cesarean section is done to deliver the baby.

Pelvic shapes
Doctors can evaluate the shape of a woman's pelvis to help predict possible problems with the baby's passage during labor and delivery. Pelvic shapes are classified into four basic types. A rounded or a long, oval pelvis usually allows for the easy passage of a baby. A narrow, heart-shaped or a flat, oval pelvis makes the baby's progress more difficult as it descends through the birth canal.

DIAGNOSING A BREECH POSITION

◆ Feeling the fetus through the woman's abdomen, the doctor finds the fetus's head under the woman's ribs and the softer buttocks and feet in the pelvic region.
◆ Using an internal (pelvic) examination, the doctor may be able to feel the fetus's buttocks.
◆ Listening through a stethoscope placed on the woman's abdomen, the doctor will hear the loudest fetal heart sounds above the woman's navel.
◆ Ultrasound scanning may be used to confirm a breech position.

POSITION OF THE BABY

During the first stage of labor, the baby is usually in a head-down position, facing the woman's back. In this position, the head is able to pass through the birth canal more easily than if the baby is in any other position. If the position of the baby is abnormal (for example, head-down but facing the woman's abdomen), the baby's head may not move down to the lowest part of the pelvis (see ENGAGEMENT on page 90) before labor begins or may move down but not pass all the way through the birth canal.

Breech position

In the early stages of pregnancy, the fetus is usually in the breech position – head upward. By the 36th week, the fetus usually has turned to a head-down position. If the fetus has not turned by week 36, it probably will not turn on its own. The doctor may try to turn the fetus so that the head is downward by manipulating the woman's abdomen (see EXTERNAL VERSION on page 73). If it can be turned easily, the fetus may change position again before delivery. There is also a risk of damaging the placenta when turning the fetus.

TYPES OF BREECH PRESENTATION AT DELIVERY

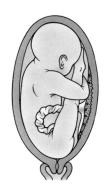

Frank breech
A baby in this presentation has his or her hips flexed and knees extended.

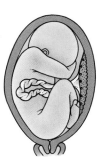

Complete breech
In this type of breech presentation, both the baby's hips and knees are flexed.

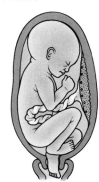

Footling breech
A footling presentation means that one or both of the baby's feet are placed over or protruding through the cervix.

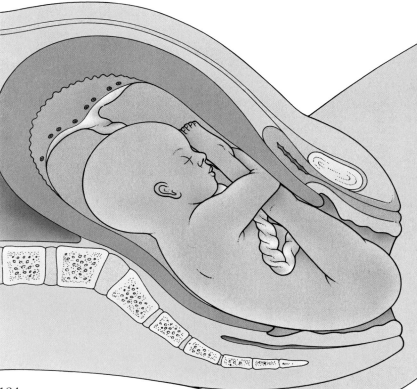

Vaginal breech delivery
A vaginal delivery may be possible for a baby in a breech presentation in some circumstances. A frank breech (see above) is the most common type of breech presentation and is usually the easiest to deliver.

Forceps delivery
When a baby in a footling breech presentation is delivered vaginally, the doctor may need to use forceps to assist the passage of the baby's head through the birth canal.

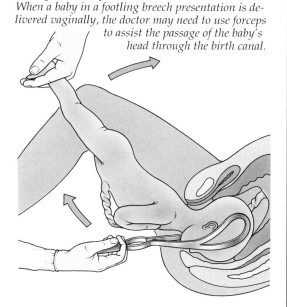

Causes of breech presentation

About 3 percent of babies are in a breech presentation at delivery. A breech presentation is more likely if there is more than one fetus, if there is an excessive amount of amniotic fluid, or if the fetus is very small. Also, if a woman has had several children, the muscles of her abdomen and uterus may have become more relaxed, enabling the fetus to more easily move into a breech position.

Delivering a breech baby

A cesarean section is done for many breech babies because of the risks to both the mother and the baby. A breech baby delivered vaginally is at increased risk of injury during birth and of receiving an insufficient supply of oxygen as a result of cord prolapse (see right).

The doctor considers a variety of factors to determine whether an attempt should be made to deliver the baby vaginally. For example, an ultrasound scan may be used to determine whether the baby is small enough to pass through the pelvis. The baby is monitored throughout labor and the doctor will be ready to perform a cesarean section if the baby shows signs of becoming stressed or if labor does not progress normally.

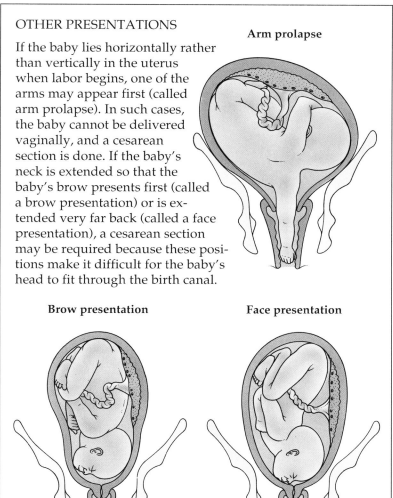

OTHER PRESENTATIONS

If the baby lies horizontally rather than vertically in the uterus when labor begins, one of the arms may appear first (called arm prolapse). In such cases, the baby cannot be delivered vaginally, and a cesarean section is done. If the baby's neck is extended so that the baby's brow presents first (called a brow presentation) or is extended very far back (called a face presentation), a cesarean section may be required because these positions make it difficult for the baby's head to fit through the birth canal.

Arm prolapse

Brow presentation

Face presentation

Cord prolapse
If the umbilical cord drops down into the cervix or the vagina (called cord prolapse), a cesarean section is necessary. To prevent compression of the cord (which could reduce the baby's oxygen supply) until the cesarean section can be performed, the doctor will have the woman get onto her hands and knees, with her head lower than her hips, and then insert his or her hand into the vagina to gently push the baby's head up and off the cord.

Prolapsed umbilical cord

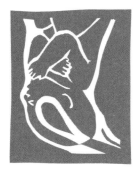

INTERVENTION DURING CHILDBIRTH

SOMETIMES IT IS **necessary** to induce labor rather than wait for it to start naturally – for example, if a woman has an illness that has been made worse because of her pregnancy or if the baby is endangered. Problems may also arise during labor that put the woman or her baby at risk and that necessitate medical intervention, such as the use of forceps or a cesarean section.

If a doctor decides to induce labor, he or she may give the woman a drug called oxytocin (see page 107). If the drug does not trigger labor or if the baby must be delivered immediately in the first stage of labor, a cesarean section will be performed. If the first stage of labor progresses, but immediate delivery is required in the second stage, the method chosen to deliver the baby will depend on the position of the baby's head and how far the baby has descended. Forceps delivery (see page 109), vacuum extraction (see page 111), or a cesarean section (see page 112) are possibilities.

INDUCING LABOR

Labor is induced only when there is a risk to the woman or to the baby if the pregnancy continues (see below). Before inducing labor, the doctor will explain to the woman why he or she recommends that labor be induced and will discuss what pain relief, if any, she would prefer (see HOW PAIN MEDICATIONS ARE GIVEN DURING LABOR AND DELIVERY on page 96). Once labor has been induced, contractions may start suddenly and be just as painful as contractions that start naturally.

WHEN IS LABOR INDUCED?

◆ If the woman develops severe preeclampsia (high blood pressure brought on by pregnancy), labor will be induced.

◆ If the pregnancy has gone beyond term, the functioning of the placenta is likely to become less efficient. Labor will be induced after week 41 or 42.

◆ If the woman has diabetes and her baby is very large or has a developmental malformation, or if the woman's diabetes is difficult to control with medication, labor will be induced early.

◆ If the baby has an abnormality and its condition is worsening, labor will be induced so that the baby can be treated.

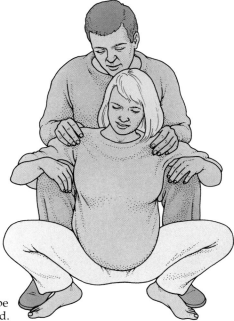

◆ If the placenta is not providing an adequate supply of oxygen and nutrients to the baby, labor will be induced.

◆ If the woman becomes Rh sensitized (see page 79) and the fetus is severely anemic and experiences heart failure, labor will be induced.

◆ If the fetus has died inside the uterus and labor has not started on its own, labor will be induced.

◆ In a multiple pregnancy (more than one fetus), if the woman develops high blood pressure, if the growth of the babies has become abnormally slow, or if the pregnancy has gone beyond week 38, labor will be induced.

METHODS FOR INDUCING LABOR

Several methods can be used to induce labor. The method chosen depends partially on whether the cervix has undergone the usual changes that occur during the last few weeks of pregnancy (see right). The baby's heart rate and the uterine contractions are monitored electronically before and during the induction of labor (see page 97).

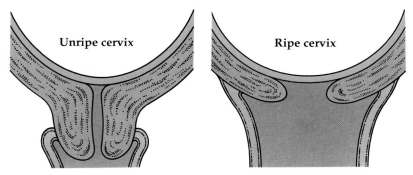

Unripe cervix

Ripe cervix

Ripening of the cervix
During the last few weeks of pregnancy, the cervix undergoes changes in preparation for labor (a process called "ripening"). The cervix becomes softer and thinner and begins to pull upward, causing its opening to widen (see above right). The more advanced this process is, the easier it is to induce labor.

Artificial rupture of the membranes

If the cervix has ripened (see above right) and has dilated at least 2 centimeters, the doctor may rupture the membranes of the amniotic sac. The doctor separates these membranes from the lower part of the uterus and then uses a special type of forceps or an amniotomy hook (shown at right) to rupture them. The release of the amniotic fluid is believed to result in the cervix producing greater amounts of substances called prostaglandins, which may stimulate contractions of the uterus. If contractions have not started after about an hour, the drug oxytocin (see below) may be given.

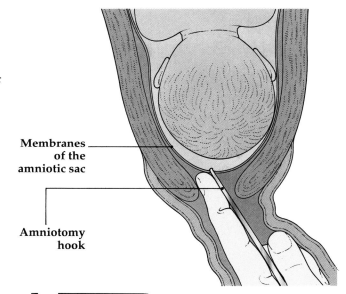

Membranes of the amniotic sac

Amniotomy hook

RISKS OF INDUCING LABOR

Artificially rupturing the membranes of the amniotic sac can cause a sudden reduction in the volume of amniotic fluid. On rare occasions, this sudden reduction of fluid can cause the placenta to separate from the wall of the uterus, depriving the baby of oxygen. The amniotic sac also serves as a natural barrier against infection. Rupturing these membranes increases the risk of infection to both the woman and the baby, although this risk does not become significant for 12 to 24 hours. If oxytocin is used to induce labor, the amount given must be carefully controlled. Too much oxytocin can cause overly strong uterine contractions that can endanger the baby.

Oxytocin infusion

Oxytocin

Oxytocin is a hormone produced by the woman's body before labor that stimulates contractions of the muscles in the uterus. If the cervix has ripened (see above), a synthetic form of oxytocin may be given by intravenous drip to induce labor. Induction is usually started slowly, with a small amount of oxytocin given while the responses of the uterus and the baby are closely monitored. The amount of oxytocin given may be gradually increased until effective contractions of the uterus start.

107

CASE HISTORY
A SMALL FETUS

Early in Laura's **pregnancy, her obstetrician noted that her blood pressure was slightly high. The obstetrician told Laura that she probably had high blood pressure before she became pregnant. As a precaution, he scheduled Laura to have her blood pressure checked twice a week. He also arranged for her to have monthly ultrasound scans, because high blood pressure can result in slowed growth of the fetus.**

PERSONAL DETAILS
Name Laura Emery
Age 22
Occupation Part-time secretary
Family Both parents are healthy; neither has high blood pressure.

MEDICAL BACKGROUND
Laura's last physical examination before she became pregnant was about 4 years ago. Laura has never had any serious health problems and she was not aware of her blood pressure ever being elevated.

THE INVESTIGATION
Laura's blood pressure remains elevated. The ultrasound scans every month are necessary to determine whether her high blood pressure is affecting the fetus. The obstetrician compares measurements of the fetus's skeleton from the scans to monitor its growth. The ultrasound scan taken at 30 weeks shows that the fetus is no longer growing as rapidly as it should.

THE DIAGNOSIS
The obstetrician tells Laura that the cause of the slowing in the growth of the fetus is a condition called PLACENTAL INSUFFICIENCY. Laura's high blood pressure has affected the blood vessels of the placenta, restricting the blood supply that carries oxygen and nutrients to the fetus. Apart from the fetus's slowed rate of growth, the obstetrician finds no other problems.

THE TREATMENT
The obstetrician tells Laura to rest in bed and says that he will continue to closely monitor her blood pressure and the growth of the fetus. He also recommends weekly monitoring of the fetus using a test called a nonstress test. He explains to Laura that, when the fetus moves, its heart rate should increase. A nonstress test checks for this increase by recording the fetus's movements and heart rate on a moving strip of paper. At week 38 of Laura's pregnancy, her obstetrician explains that the reduced supply of oxygen is now posing too great a risk to the fetus and he recommends that labor be induced.

THE OUTCOME
Laura is admitted to the hospital and monitoring of the fetus's heartbeat is started immediately. The obstetrician induces labor by giving the drug oxytocin by intravenous drip. It takes a while for Laura's contractions to become regular but, once they do, her labor is relatively short and she gives birth to a baby girl.

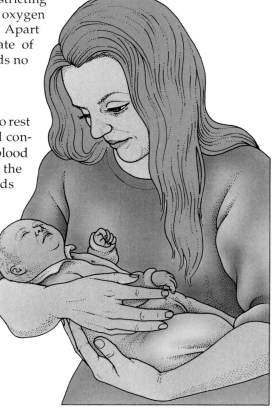

Small but healthy
Although Laura's new daughter is small, the obstetrician assures Laura that, with proper nourishment, the baby should grow and develop at a normal rate.

FORCEPS DELIVERY

Obstetrical forceps (a pair of spoonlike instruments) can be inserted into the woman's vagina during a difficult labor to help deliver the head of a baby. In some cases the first stage of labor progresses without any problems, but, during the second stage, immediate delivery is necessary because of a possible risk to either the woman or the baby. If the baby's head has descended into the lower part of the woman's pelvis, the doctor may be able to deliver the baby with the help of forceps (see page 110).

In most cases, a forceps delivery is quicker and less traumatic than a cesarean section and is less dangerous for the woman and the baby. However, there are some risks involved in a forceps delivery. Forceps may leave temporary marks on the baby's head, put stress on the baby's neck and spine, or damage nerves in the baby's face. Possible risks to the woman include tearing of the tissues of the vagina or temporary retention of urine as a result of the tissue injury caused by the use of forceps.

When are forceps used?

The doctor may use forceps to deliver a baby in the following situations:

◆ If changes in the baby's heart rate indicate the baby is stressed.

◆ If contractions and pushing during the second stage of labor are no longer effectively moving the baby down through the birth canal.

◆ If the woman is exhausted and no longer able to push effectively.

◆ If the woman has a medical problem (such as heart disease) that makes the stress of pushing during the second stage of labor dangerous for her.

◆ During a breech birth (see page 104) to deliver the baby's head.

Pain medication

When forceps are used, either a regional anesthetic (an epidural) or a local anesthetic (a pudendal block) will be given. If epidural anesthesia is already being administered (see page 96), additional anesthesia can be given through the catheter if necessary. Otherwise, a pudendal block, which numbs the vagina and surrounding tissues, will be given.

WHEN IS A FORCEPS DELIVERY SAFE?

For a forceps delivery to be done safely, all of the following conditions must be present: the cervix must be fully dilated (see page 94); the membranes of the amniotic sac must be ruptured; the widest diameter of the baby's head must be engaged (see ENGAGEMENT on page 90) and be in or near the lower part of the pelvis; the doctor must be absolutely certain of the position of the baby's head; the pelvis must be wide enough for the baby's head to pass through safely; and the woman's bladder must be empty.

EPISIOTOMY

An episiotomy is an incision made in the woman's perineum (the tissue between the vaginal opening and the anus) to prevent tearing of the perineum and the vagina or injury to the baby's head. An episiotomy may be performed when the vaginal tissues have not stretched adequately to allow passage of the baby's head; during delivery of a premature baby to avoid pressure on the baby's head; or when forceps must be used to deliver the baby. After the placenta has been delivered, the episiotomy incision is closed with dissolvable stitches. The area around the incision will be sore for a few days. Applying an ice pack, taking a warm sitz bath (sitting in a shallow tub of water), or sitting on a pillow or an inflated tube may help relieve the discomfort. To avoid possible infection, pour or squirt warm water over the area each time you urinate or have a bowel movement and then carefully pat the area dry.

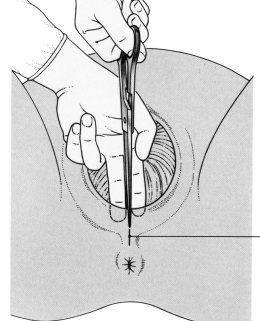

Incision

Making the incision
An anesthetic is injected along the line where the episiotomy incision will be made. The doctor then inserts two fingers against the back wall of the vagina to protect the baby's head. During a contraction, scissors are used to make the incision between the vaginal opening and the anus.

FORCEPS DELIVERY

Although forceps are no longer used as often as they were in the past, they are sometimes necessary to deliver a baby. Talk to your doctor about when he or she recommends using forceps and the risks involved in a forceps delivery (see page 109). The procedure used for a forceps delivery is described below.

3 The doctor checks to see that no vaginal tissue is caught between the forceps blades. He or she checks the position of the blades on the baby's head and then locks the handles of the two blades together.

1 The doctor inserts the fingers of one hand into the woman's vagina. He or she then slips one of the forceps blades into the vagina, using the other hand to guide the blade along the side of the baby's head.

Handles of forceps

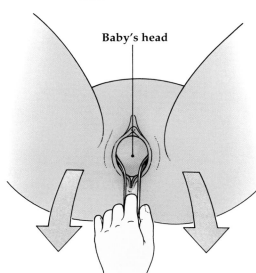

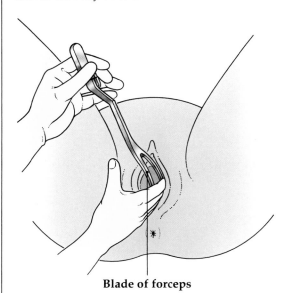

Blade of forceps

4 The doctor gently pulls downward on the forceps. As the baby's head descends, the doctor shifts the gentle pulling to a more horizontal and then upward direction. The doctor coordinates his or her pulling action with the woman's pushing efforts and contractions. As the delivery becomes imminent, an episiotomy (see page 109) is done.

Baby's head

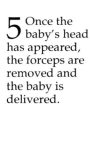

2 The doctor inserts the other blade of the forceps into the vagina.

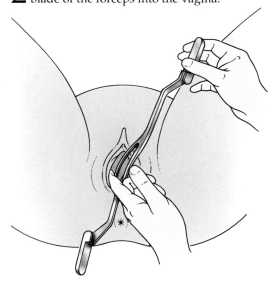

5 Once the baby's head has appeared, the forceps are removed and the baby is delivered.

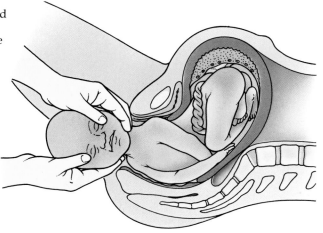

DELIVERY BY VACUUM EXTRACTION

Vacuum extraction, a technique developed in the 1950s, is sometimes used as an alternative to forceps to assist in delivery of a baby (see below).

The circumstances in which vacuum extraction is used are generally the same as those for the use of forceps – if progress during the second stage of labor stops, if the woman has a medical condition (such as heart disease) that could make the continuation of labor dangerous for her, if the woman is exhausted and can no longer push effectively, or if the baby begins to show signs of stress. Vacuum extraction is not used if the baby's face or brow is presenting (see page 105), if the baby is premature, or if the baby is severely stressed.

Vacuum extraction often requires less pain medication than is needed for the use of forceps and does not necessarily require that an episiotomy be done. However, there are some risks to both the woman and the baby. These risks are possible cuts and bruising of the baby's scalp or bleeding inside the baby's skull and possible injury to tissues of the woman's vagina and cervix. The suction used with this technique may cause the baby's scalp to swell, but the swelling usually goes away soon after delivery.

HOW VACUUM EXTRACTION IS PERFORMED

A vacuum extractor consists of a disc-shaped plastic cup that is attached to a vacuum pump. Delivery by vacuum extraction is generally slower than with forceps, but poses less risk of damage to the woman's genital tract.

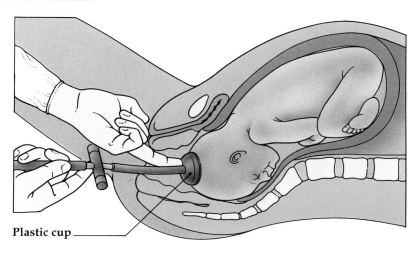

1 The plastic cup is inserted into the woman's vagina and applied to the baby's head. When the vacuum pump is turned on, the suction created by the pump holds the cup in place on the baby's head.

Plastic cup

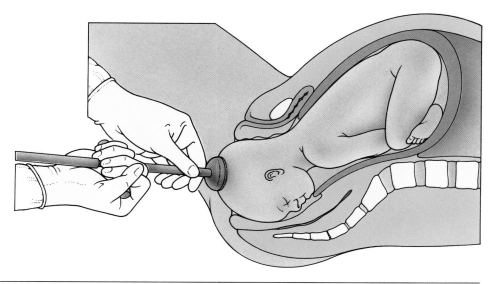

2 Using the handle that is attached to the plastic cup, the doctor gently pulls with each contraction, until the baby's head appears at the opening of the vagina. If necessary, an episiotomy is performed to deliver the baby. After the head appears, the doctor turns off the vacuum pump and removes the cup from the baby's head. The baby is then delivered.

CESAREAN SECTION

A cesarean section is a surgical procedure done to deliver the baby through an incision in the woman's abdomen. This procedure is believed to have been performed as early as the 16th century. In the past, the rate of death for women who had cesarean sections was very high. The safety of a cesarean section has increased dramatically over the years as a result of refined surgical techniques (see right) and advances in medical technology. Since the development and use of blood transfusions, antibiotic drugs, and new types of anesthetics, cesarean section has become a safe procedure. However, on rare occasions, it is still a cause of death (in less than one per 1,000 women).

Types of incisions for a cesarean section
In the past, a vertical incision in the upper (muscular) part of the uterus was used for a cesarean section. Doctors now usually use a horizontal incision in the lower (fibrous) part of the uterus, which is thinner and contains fewer blood vessels than the upper part. The site of a previous incision in the lower part of the uterus is under much less strain and is much less likely to rupture during a subsequent normal labor than one in the upper part of the uterus.

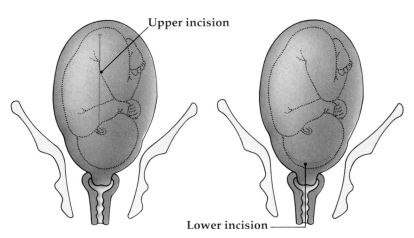

Upper incision

Lower incision

WHEN IS A CESAREAN SECTION PERFORMED?

About one fourth of births in the US today are by cesarean section. A cesarean section may be scheduled (if the doctor determines that the risks of labor and a vaginal delivery are too high) or be done as an emergency procedure if problems develop during labor. You should discuss with your doctor his or her feelings about when a cesarean section may be necessary. Some indicators that a cesarean section may be necessary are listed below.

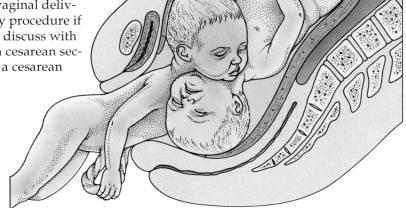

Problems for the woman
◆ Failure of labor to progress from the first to the second stage
◆ Unsuccessful attempts to induce labor
◆ Rapidly worsening preeclampsia (high blood pressure brought on by pregnancy), in which it is not possible to induce labor
◆ Two or more previous cesarean sections
◆ Scarring of the uterus from previous surgery (for example, for removal of fibroids)
◆ An active outbreak of genital herpes infection (which could be transmitted to the baby if he or she is delivered vaginally)

Problems for the baby
◆ Stress caused by a lack of oxygen
◆ Protrusion of the umbilical cord into the cervix or vagina (called cord prolapse)
◆ Twin birth if the first baby to be delivered is in a breech presentation
◆ Multiple birth (usually for triplets or more)
◆ Horizontal or other presentations of the baby that make vaginal delivery impossible
◆ A very large baby

Locked twins
In rare instances, the chins of twins may interlock, so that neither twin can move into a position to be delivered vaginally. A cesarean section is necessary.

Problems for the woman and baby
◆ A baby whose head is too large to pass through the woman's pelvis
◆ Abnormally low positioning of the placenta in the uterus or detachment of the placenta from the wall of the uterus
◆ Unsuccessful forceps delivery

DELIVERY AFTER A CESAREAN

After having a cesarean section, 60 to 80 percent of women can deliver a subsequent baby vaginally. A vaginal delivery may be possible if the incision for the earlier cesarean was made horizontally in the lower part of the uterus.

CASE HISTORY
WEAK CONTRACTIONS

LESLIE'S PREGNANCY HAD PROGRESSED **normally and she had not experienced any problems. When labor started, everything appeared to be happening as it should. Leslie called her doctor when the contractions started occurring about every 10 minutes. The doctor told her that she should come to the hospital.**

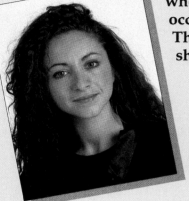

PERSONAL DETAILS
Name Leslie Parsons
Age 23
Occupation Illustrator
Family Both of Leslie's parents are healthy.

MEDICAL BACKGROUND
Throughout Leslie's prenatal visits, her blood pressure and the results of her urine and blood tests have been normal, and she has not had a problem with retention of fluids. The baby has developed normally and Leslie has felt good.

AT THE HOSPITAL
Leslie's doctor does frequent internal (pelvic) examinations to check the amount of dilation (widening) of the cervix. He assures Leslie that everything looks fine so far. But when her cervix has dilated to about 4 centimeters, Leslie's contractions begin to weaken and the cervix does not dilate any farther.

THE DIAGNOSIS
Leslie's doctor explains that she is having INEFFECTIVE CONTRACTIONS. This means that the contractions are no longer strong enough to fully dilate the cervix. He tells Leslie that the cause of this problem is not fully understood but that it may be possible to stimulate her contractions.

THE TREATMENT
Leslie's doctor gives her the drug oxytocin by intravenous drip to try to stimulate more effective contractions. The contractions and the baby's heart rate are closely monitored (see below). Leslie's contractions get stronger but after more than 2 hours the doctor notes that the cervix has not dilated any more and that the baby's head has not descended any farther into Leslie's pelvis. Leslie's doctor explains to her that it is highly unlikely her cervix will dilate any more. He recommends that a cesarean section be done. After asking many questions, Leslie agrees to have the operation.

Leslie is given a general anesthetic and a cesarean section is done. A healthy baby girl is delivered.

THE OUTCOME
Leslie recovers without complications and she and her new daughter are able to go home in a few days. At a follow-up visit to her doctor, Leslie asks him if she will be able to have a vaginal delivery if she has another baby. The doctor assures Leslie that, because the incision was made in the lower part of her uterus, there is no reason why she should not be able to attempt to deliver future babies vaginally.

Internal monitoring of the baby
An electrode is inserted into Leslie's vagina and attached to the baby's scalp so that the baby's heartbeat can be continuously monitored. A pressure-sensitive catheter (thin tube) is inserted into her uterus next to the baby to monitor the contractions.

Scalp electrode   Pressure-sensitive catheter

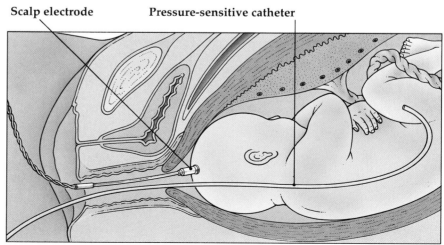

SURGICAL PROCEDURES
CESAREAN SECTION

A CESAREAN SECTION **is performed in an operating room that is often adjacent to the labor and delivery area. If the doctor knows in advance that a cesarean will be performed (for example, if the woman is having triplets or has already had two previous cesareans), the operation is usually done at around week 39. If an epidural anesthetic (which is regional) rather than a general anesthetic is used, the woman's partner is often allowed to be present to provide support. The actual delivery of the baby takes only a few minutes, but the entire procedure takes 40 to 60 minutes.**

1 The lower part of the woman's abdomen is shaved and a catheter (thin tube) is inserted into the bladder to drain any urine. An intravenous infusion of fluids is started. An epidural (see page 96) or a general anesthetic is given. An epidural anesthetic carries less risk, but general anesthesia – which takes effect more quickly – may be needed (for example, if vaginal bleeding is heavy).

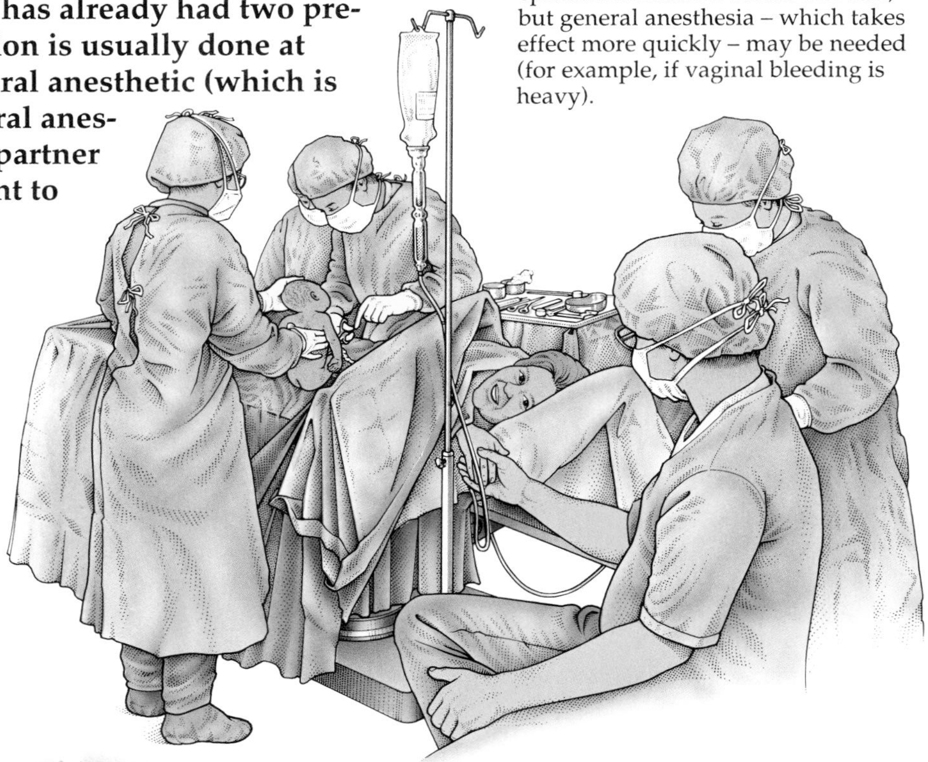

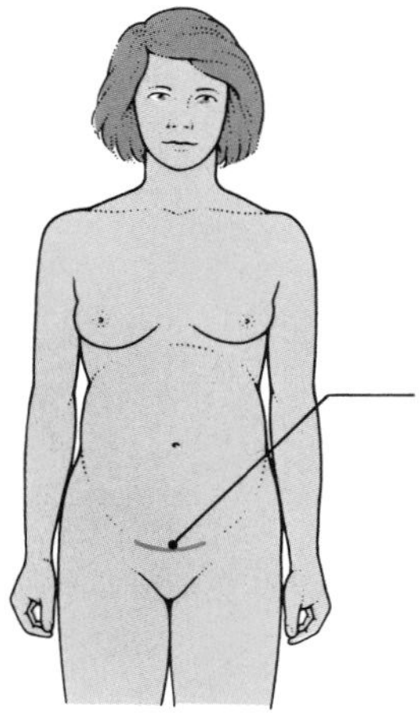

Incision

2 On the operating table, the woman is tilted slightly onto one side. Her abdomen is cleaned with antiseptic solutions and sterile cloths are applied, leaving the lower part of the abdomen exposed. The doctor makes a horizontal incision, usually near the pubic hairline. Occasionally, a vertical incision (which extends from just below the navel to the pubic hairline) is used.

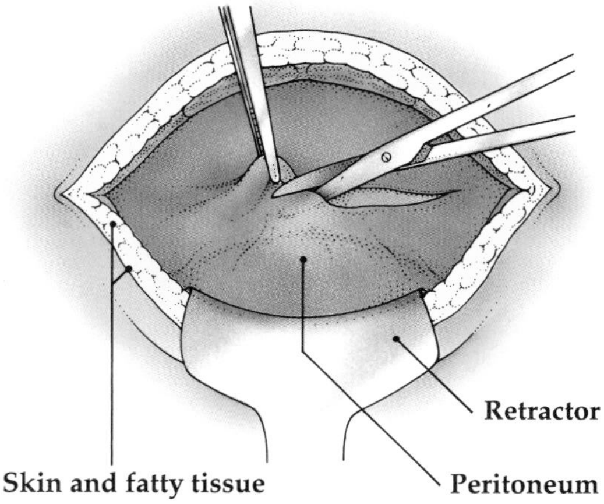

Skin and fatty tissue

Retractor

Peritoneum

3 The doctor deepens the incision, carefully cutting through the skin and fatty tissues of the abdominal wall and places a retractor in the lower edge of the incision to hold the tissues back. He or she then makes a horizontal incision in the thin membrane called the peritoneum that covers the abdominal cavity.

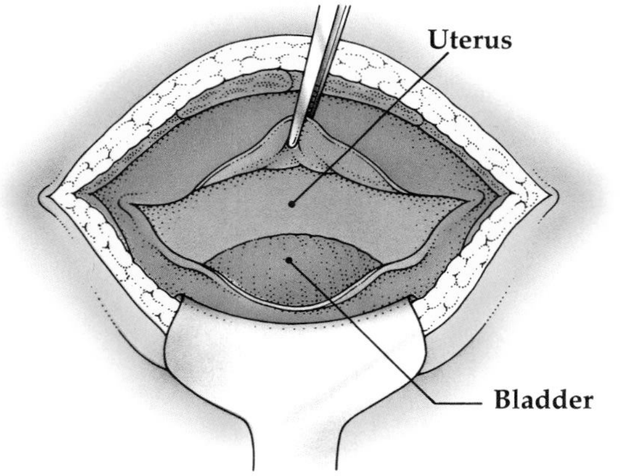

Uterus

Bladder

4 The doctor cuts through fibrous tissue inside the abdominal cavity to move the top part of the bladder away from the uterus.

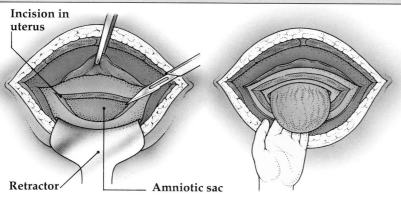

Incision in uterus

Retractor   Amniotic sac

5 The retractor is repositioned to hold the bladder out of the way. The doctor makes a horizontal incision in the lower part of the uterus down to the membranes of the amniotic sac covering the baby.

6 The doctor ruptures the membranes and inserts a hand below the baby's head. The baby is removed from the uterus by gently pulling his or her head upward.

7 An intravenous injection of oxytocin is given to make the uterus contract and stop any bleeding. The baby's mouth and nose are cleared. The cord is clamped and cut, and the doctor removes the placenta and the amniotic sac from the uterus.

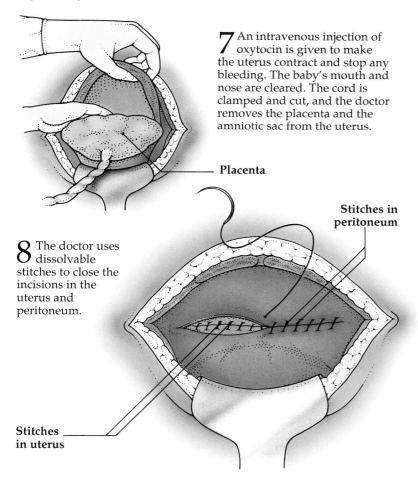

Placenta

Stitches in peritoneum

8 The doctor uses dissolvable stitches to close the incisions in the uterus and peritoneum.

Stitches in uterus

9 The incision in the abdomen is closed with either small metal clips (called staples) or stitches. A large adhesive bandage is applied to the incision. The catheter and the intravenous drip are usually left in overnight. An antibiotic is sometimes given through the intravenous drip to reduce the chances of infection.

10 The woman is usually able to go home after 3 to 4 days.

ASK YOUR DOCTOR
EFFECTS OF INTERVENTION

Q I have heard that forceps can permanently damage the baby's head. Is this true?

A Forceps only rarely cause any permanent damage to the baby's head. Sometimes the forceps leave slight, temporary marks on the baby's face, but these marks fade quickly. A doctor carefully evaluates the risks of using forceps and, if he or she has any doubt that forceps can be used safely, a cesarean section is performed instead.

Q My sister had to have a blood transfusion after she had a cesarean section. Is this a routine procedure after a cesarean? How about after a vaginal delivery?

A In most cases, a blood transfusion is not necessary after a cesarean section or a vaginal delivery. Blood transfusions are given only if the woman has had excessive bleeding after either type of delivery and if the doctor thinks that the amount of blood that was lost could place her life in danger.

Q I have gone a week past my due date and my doctor says she will have to induce labor if I don't go into labor soon. I had planned to have a natural childbirth. Will this still be possible if my labor has to be induced?

A Yes. Your doctor is probably concerned that if your baby grows much larger a vaginal delivery may not be possible. Inducing labor is just a way of getting contractions started if labor does not start on its own. This procedure should not affect how you deliver the baby, but the contractions may be strong even in the early stages of labor.

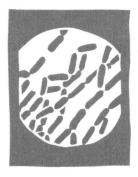

POSSIBLE COMPLICATIONS OF CHILDBIRTH

O CCASIONALLY, COMPLICATIONS DEVELOP during or after the birth of a baby. Your doctor will watch for warning signs of complications during labor and delivery. After you are home, you should be alert to signs that tell you to call your doctor so that possible problems can be diagnosed and treated promptly.

After childbirth, a woman should let her doctor know immediately if she has any unusual symptoms such as heavy vaginal bleeding or a fever.

VAGINAL BLEEDING

Some bleeding from the vagina after childbirth is normal. After the baby has been delivered, contractions of the muscles of the uterus cause the placenta to separate from the wall of the uterus. After the placenta has been expelled, these muscles continue to contract. The contractions cause the blood vessels of the uterus that supplied the placenta to close. As a result, the amount of vaginal bleeding gradually decreases and usually stops within 5 to 6 weeks after delivery. If this process does not progress normally, excessive bleeding may occur. Heavy vaginal bleeding within the first 24 hours after delivery is an uncommon complication but can be life-threatening if it is not treated promptly. Call your doctor immediately if you have any signs of abnormal vaginal bleeding.

Causes of excessive bleeding

Tearing of genital tissues or rupture of the wall of the uterus can cause excessive bleeding immediately after delivery (see INJURY TO GENITAL TISSUES on page 118). Excessive bleeding can also occur if the placenta or parts of it remain in the uterus or if the uterus does not contract after the placenta is delivered (see CONTROLLING BLEEDING on page 117). Heavy vaginal bleeding that starts more than 24 hours after delivery may be caused by a fragment of the placenta that has remained in the uterus or by an infection in the uterus (see INFECTION on page 120).

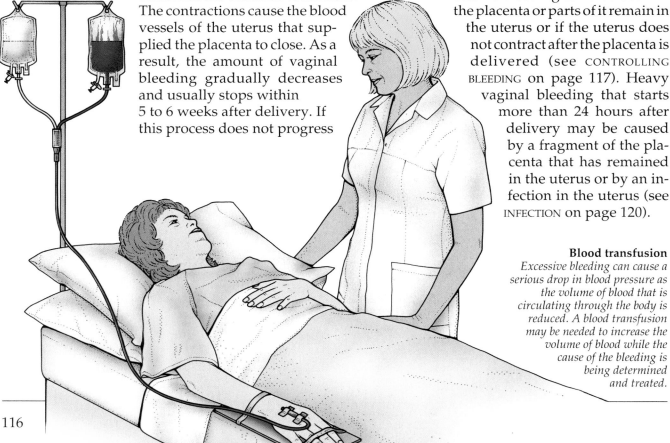

Blood transfusion
Excessive bleeding can cause a serious drop in blood pressure as the volume of blood that is circulating through the body is reduced. A blood transfusion may be needed to increase the volume of blood while the cause of the bleeding is being determined and treated.

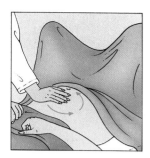

Massaging the abdomen
If contractions are not strong enough to control bleeding, the doctor may try to stimulate the uterine muscles by using a circular, massaging motion on the woman's abdomen.

Controlling bleeding

Excessive bleeding sometimes occurs because the uterus does not contract after delivery of the placenta. This problem may occur after a long labor because the muscles of the uterus are no longer able to contract. It may also occur if the uterus has been overstretched because of an excessive amount of amniotic fluid, a very large baby, a multiple birth, or several previous deliveries. Vaginal bleeding may also be excessive if the placenta was attached to the lower part of the uterus. The contractions in the lower part of the uterus are not as strong as contractions in the upper part and may not be adequate to close the blood vessels where the placenta was attached.

To stop the bleeding, the doctor will try to stimulate contractions by massaging the abdomen (see above) and giving the drug oxytocin (see page 107).

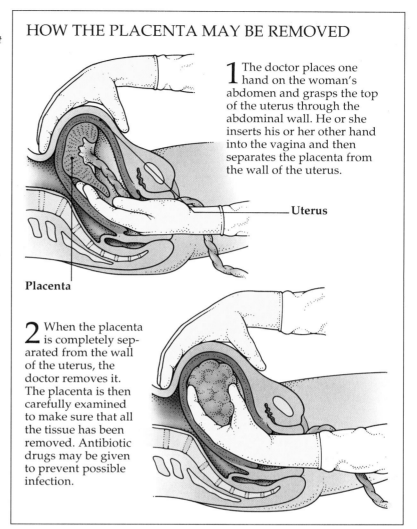

HOW THE PLACENTA MAY BE REMOVED

1 The doctor places one hand on the woman's abdomen and grasps the top of the uterus through the abdominal wall. He or she inserts his or her other hand into the vagina and then separates the placenta from the wall of the uterus.

Uterus

Placenta

2 When the placenta is completely separated from the wall of the uterus, the doctor removes it. The placenta is then carefully examined to make sure that all the tissue has been removed. Antibiotic drugs may be given to prevent possible infection.

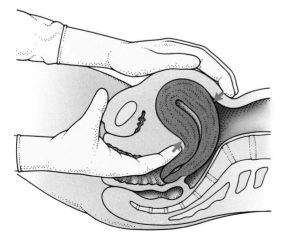

Compression of the uterus to control bleeding
Until the amount of oxytocin being given is sufficient to control bleeding, the doctor may compress the uterus between one hand placed inside the woman's vagina and the other hand on her abdomen.

Removing the placenta

If the natural contractions of the uterine muscles are not strong enough, the placenta may not be expelled or part of the placenta may not separate from the wall of the uterus. Fragments of tissue from the placenta that remain in the uterus can prevent further uterine contractions that are necessary to close the blood vessels. To help deliver the placenta, the drug oxytocin will be given to try to stimulate contractions. If this treatment is not successful, the doctor will give the woman painkilling medication and then remove the placenta (see above). The technique described above is also used to remove any fragments of the placenta that remain in the uterus.

INVERTED UTERUS

In rare cases, pulling on the umbilical cord to remove the placenta when it is still attached to the wall of the uterus can turn the uterus inside out – the top of the uterus is pulled down through the vagina (known as an inverted uterus). Using a general anesthetic, the doctor pushes the uterus back up through the vagina.

First-degree tear
A first-degree tear involves the labia and the mucous membrane of the vagina. This type of tear often heals on its own or may require one or two stitches.

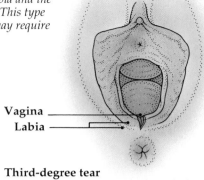

Vagina
Labia

Second-degree tear
A second-degree tear is a tear into the muscles of the perineum (between the vaginal opening and the anus). The doctor will inject a local anesthetic and close this type of tear with stitches.

Third-degree tear
A third-degree tear extends through the anal sphincter (the muscle that keeps the anus closed). This type of tear must be carefully repaired with stitches to ensure that the sphincter muscle is not weakened.

INJURY TO GENITAL TISSUES

The tissues that are injured most commonly during childbirth are those between the opening of the vagina and the anus (called the perineum). Tears of the perineal tissues are more common in a woman who is having her first child because these tissues have not been stretched during a previous delivery. A tear is classified according to its severity (see left and below).

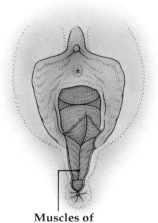

Muscles of perineum

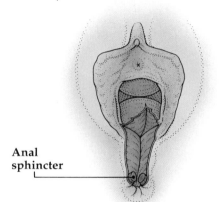

Anal sphincter

Fourth-degree tear
A fourth-degree tear extends from the vagina through to the rectum. The torn tissues are carefully stitched together layer by layer to minimize any chance of stool leaking into the vagina and to ensure that the woman can control passage of stool. Medication is often given to keep the stool soft until the tear has healed.

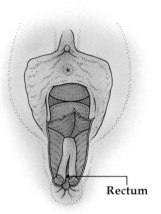

Rectum

IS AN EPISIOTOMY NECESSARY?

An episiotomy is an incision made in the perineum (the tissue between the vaginal opening and the anus) that allows the baby's head to be delivered more easily. An episiotomy is done in about 90 percent of deliveries. There is continuing controversy about the risks and benefits and the need for episiotomies. You should discuss this subject with your doctor.

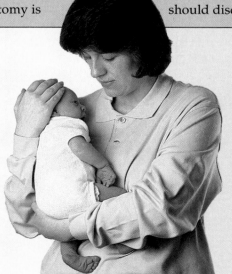

Reasons for performing an episiotomy
◆ An episiotomy prevents a ragged tear in the perineum.
◆ An episiotomy incision is easier to repair than a tear.
◆ An episiotomy may be done to deliver a stressed baby quickly.
◆ Possible brain damage, caused by pressure on the baby's head, is prevented. A premature baby is especially prone to injury during delivery.
◆ A woman is able to deliver a large baby or a breech baby more easily.
◆ Forceps can be used more safely and easily.

Reasons against performing an episiotomy
◆ A tear in the perineal tissues is usually not as long as an episiotomy incision.
◆ More bleeding occurs with an episiotomy than with a tear.
◆ An episiotomy incision can be stitched shut too tightly, causing discomfort after it heals.
◆ An episiotomy may cause pain as the incision heals.
◆ Sexual intercourse may be uncomfortable for longer after a delivery involving an episiotomy.

Hematoma

As a result of internal bleeding from a blood vessel, blood may collect in the tissues around the vagina. This localized collection of blood is called a hematoma. If the hematoma is small, it may be reabsorbed on its own. A large hematoma can cause severe pain; surgery may be needed to drain it.

Tearing of the cervix

In rare cases, the cervix may be injured during labor. The tissues of the cervix may tear if labor proceeds very rapidly or if forceps are used. A tear will be closed with stitches to prevent problems in a future pregnancy, such as cervical incompetence (inability of the cervix to remain closed during pregnancy).

Repairing a torn cervix
A tear in the cervix can often be repaired without an anesthetic; if necessary, the doctor will inject the tissues with a local anesthetic (see page 51). The doctor grasps the cervix with forceps and pulls it down into the vagina, then stitches the tear closed.

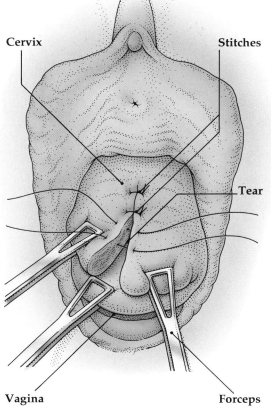

Ruptured uterus
Rupture of the uterus is rare. It is usually the result of rupture of a scar from a previous cesarean section, particularly if the cesarean section was done using an incision in the upper part of the uterus (see page 112). A scar from a cesarean section in the lower part of the uterus is unlikely to rupture. If the uterus ruptures, a cesarean section is done immediately. A tear in the uterus can usually be closed with stitches. In rare cases, a hysterectomy is necessary.

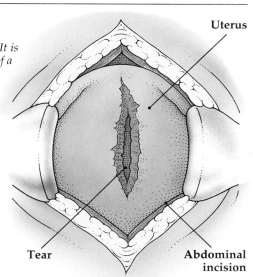

BLOOD CLOTS

A woman who has recently had a baby can develop a blood clot in the deep veins in her legs (called deep vein thrombosis) as a result of decreased circulation through these veins. The decreased circulation may be caused by a lower level of physical activity or by the pressure that the enlarged uterus puts on the veins that carry blood from the legs. A piece of a blood clot that has formed in the legs may break away and move through the bloodstream into the lungs, where it can block a blood vessel. This blockage, called a pulmonary embolism, can be life-threatening.

A small blood clot usually dissolves gradually; injections of the drug heparin may be given to prevent more clots from forming. A large blood clot may be treated with drugs to dissolve it; in some cases, surgery is necessary to remove the clot.

Preventing deep vein thrombosis
To prevent deep vein thrombosis, a woman is encouraged to get up and move around as early as possible after delivery.

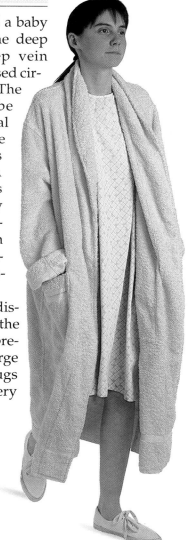

INFECTION

Infection occurring after an uncomplicated delivery is rare. Many women will have a low fever for the first few days after delivery, but body temperature usually spontaneously returns to normal. A fever on the third or fourth day could be a sign of infection; treatment with an antibiotic drug may be needed. Signs and symptoms vary, depending on the site of the infection (see below).

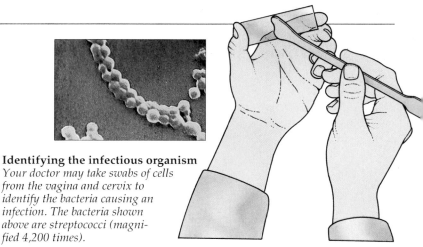

Identifying the infectious organism
Your doctor may take swabs of cells from the vagina and cervix to identify the bacteria causing an infection. The bacteria shown above are streptococci (magnified 4,200 times).

Signs of infection
It is important that you be alert to possible signs of infection. If you notice any of the signs indicated below, contact your doctor immediately.

Pain in the lower part of the abdomen may be a sign of infection in the uterus, especially if the pain persists and worsens.

Painful urination or difficulty urinating may indicate a urinary tract infection.

Foul-smelling vaginal discharge may mean you have an infection of the genital tract.

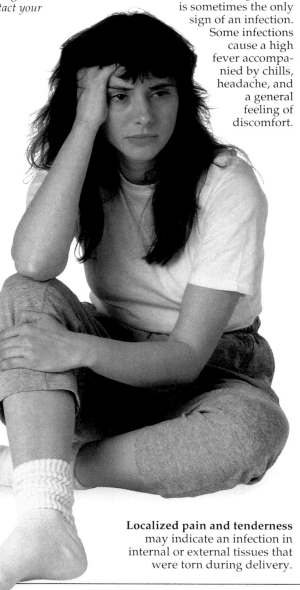

Slight fever is sometimes the only sign of an infection. Some infections cause a high fever accompanied by chills, headache, and a general feeling of discomfort.

Localized pain and tenderness may indicate an infection in internal or external tissues that were torn during delivery.

Infection of the genital tract

Infection of the genital tract may be caused by bacteria from inside or outside the body. In rare cases, bacteria that live harmlessly within the vagina may cause infection if the mucous membranes of the vagina have been injured during childbirth. After childbirth, infection is likely if a fragment of tissue from the placenta remains in the uterus.

If your doctor suspects you have an infection, he or she will take swabs from the cervix and vagina so that the infectious organism can be identified (see above). Treatment with a broad-spectrum antibiotic (a drug that is effective against a wide range of bacteria) is started immediately. When the type of bacterium is identified, the antibiotic can be changed to fight the specific infection.

If an internal examination shows that the uterus is enlarged and the cervix has remained open, an ultrasound scan may be done to check for placental tissue. If the scan shows placental tissue in the uterus, the doctor will scrape the uterine lining (a procedure called curettage) to remove the remaining tissue.

Urinary tract infection

Inserting a catheter (a thin tube) into the bladder to drain urine during labor increases the risk of infection of the urinary tract. If your doctor suspects that you have developed a urinary tract infection after delivery, a sample of your urine may be tested and antibiotics given.

CASE HISTORY
ABNORMAL BLEEDING

CAROLINE WAS IN THE **delivery room giving birth to her third child. Her labor had been fairly short and there were no serious problems during the delivery of the baby – a healthy baby girl weighing almost 8 pounds. However, Caroline experienced an excessive amount of vaginal bleeding before the placenta was expelled. The obstetrician performed an internal examination to determine the cause of the bleeding.**

PERSONAL DETAILS
Name Caroline Weinmann
Age 33
Occupation Accountant
Family Caroline's two sons are healthy.

MEDICAL BACKGROUND
Caroline has not had any serious health problems. Her previous pregnancies and deliveries were normal.

THE EXAMINATION
During the internal examination, the obstetrician does not find any tears in the cervix or vagina and notes that the uterus seems to be contracting normally. Caroline's blood pressure and pulse rate are normal. A blood test shows that her level of hemoglobin (the oxygen-carrying part of red blood cells) is also normal.

Caroline's condition is closely monitored and, after 20 minutes, the placenta is expelled. The obstetrician carefully examines the placenta and finds that fragments of tissue are missing. Because Caroline's blood pressure, pulse rate, and hemoglobin levels are still normal, he decides to wait to see if the uterus will continue to contract and if the remaining tissues will be expelled. But, after a short time, no more placental tissue is expelled and the vaginal bleeding continues.

THE DIAGNOSIS
The obstetrician tells Caroline that the vaginal bleeding is the result of RETAINED PLACENTAL TISSUE. He explains to her that an empty uterus contracts to close the blood vessels in the wall of the uterus where the placenta was attached. If part of the placenta remains in the uterus, the uterus cannot contract adequately and bleeding continues.

THE TREATMENT
The obstetrician tells Caroline that he will have to remove the placental tissue. After giving Caroline a pain-killing medication, the obstetrician inserts his hand into her uterus, carefully separates all the fragments of placental tissue from the uterine wall, and removes them. The bleeding increases in the first few minutes after the tissues have been removed, and then the uterus contracts and the bleeding stops.

THE OUTCOME
Although Caroline's hemoglobin level has dropped, the obstetrician decides that a blood transfusion is not necessary. He explains to Caroline that the decreased level of hemoglobin is not serious and that her body's blood cell manufacturing mechanism will quickly make up the deficit. The obstetrician recommends that Caroline start taking iron, which is essential to the formation of hemoglobin. Although she feels very weak and tired, Caroline tells the obstetrician that she is relieved that her baby is healthy and that she is going to be fine.

The next day, Caroline feels much stronger. The obstetrician tells her she can go home the following day. At her 6-week checkup, a blood test shows that Caroline's hemoglobin level has returned to normal.

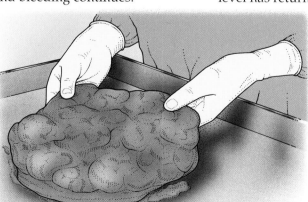

Examining the placenta
After the placenta has been delivered, it is carefully examined to ensure that all the tissues have been expelled from the uterus.

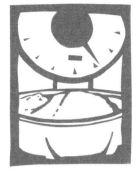

YOUR NEWBORN BABY

PARENTS ANTICIPATE their first moments holding their newborn baby with great excitement. Often the parents have formed unrealistic pictures in their minds about what their son or daughter will look like and are unprepared when they see their newborn baby for the first time. Don't be surprised or worried if your baby does not look, behave, or respond as you had expected.

Among the many questions and concerns racing through new parents' minds is, of course, whether their baby is healthy. You can be assured that a wide range of tests and measurements will be done to assess your baby's health.

WHAT YOUR NEWBORN BABY WILL LOOK LIKE

A newborn baby usually weighs between 5 ½ and 9 pounds. Soon after birth, the baby will lose up to 10 percent of his or her birth weight but will gain the weight back by about the 10th day. On average, a newborn baby is 20 inches long.

Your baby's head

Your baby's head may look large in relation to the rest of his or her body and may appear misshapen. This unusual shape results from the pressure on the soft bones of the skull as the baby passes through the birth canal. The shape of the baby's head becomes more natural within about 2 weeks. The baby's scalp has two soft areas over gaps (called fontanelles) between bones of the skull.

Your baby may have a headful of hair or none at all. Fine, downy hair (called lanugo) may cover the baby's shoulders, back, forehead, and temples; this hair will fall out during the first month.

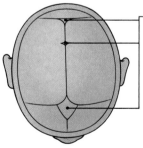

Fontanelles are gaps between the skull bones that have not yet joined together. By about 18 months, these bones will have closed over the soft areas.

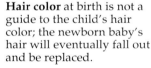

Hair color at birth is not a guide to the child's hair color; the newborn baby's hair will eventually fall out and be replaced.

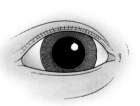

Eye color is often gray-blue, but may change gradually over the next few months.

Breathing may be irregular – fast, slow, shallow, or deep. Hiccups are common.

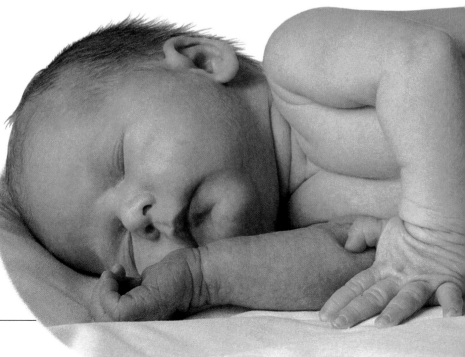

APGAR SCORE

Virginia Apgar, an American doctor, devised a scoring system to assess the condition of a newborn baby during the first few minutes after birth. Five features are evaluated and scored on a scale of 0 to 2 – the highest possible total score is 10. The Apgar score is taken at 1 minute and at 5 minutes after birth. This score helps the doctor evaluate whether the baby needs any immediate special attention. Sometimes babies who have been through a long labor or a stressful delivery will have low Apgar scores. The Apgar score is not designed to (nor can it) measure a baby's long-term potential or development. Most babies develop normally even if their Apgar score at birth was relatively low.

SIGN	SCORE		
	0	1	2
Heart rate	Absent	Less than 100 beats per minute	More than 100 beats per minute
Breathing pattern and crying	Absent	Weak cry, irregular breathing	Strong cry, regular breathing
Skin color*	Blue or pale	Pink body, blue extremities	All pink
Muscle tone	Limp	Some bending of arms and legs	Active bending of arms and legs
Reflex response (tested by inserting a thin tube into the baby's nose)	None	Grimace	Cry

*For nonwhite infants, skin color is scored by examining the inside of the mouth and the lips, the whites of the eyes, the palms of the hands, and the soles of the feet.

"ROOMING-IN"

Some hospitals offer a family-oriented option in maternity care called "rooming-in." Rooming-in allows the woman to keep her baby in her hospital room (the father can stay overnight too). If the woman becomes too tired, the baby can be taken to the nursery for a few hours. Although rooming-in may not be right for everyone, many first-time parents find it is a wonderful way to get acquainted with their newborn. If they need help or have a question, the nurses are right down the hall.

The stump of the umbilical cord usually dries up and falls off within 10 days. Redness around the stump may indicate an infection.

Peeling of the skin, particularly the skin on the baby's hands and feet, is common during the first week.

Examining the newborn baby
Immediately after birth, a doctor or nurse will assess the baby's condition, rating it according to the Apgar scoring system (see above). He or she will also look for any obvious abnormality. For healthy-looking babies, a complete physical examination is done within 24 hours. If there is reason to suspect a problem, a pediatrician may be called in to examine the baby immediately.

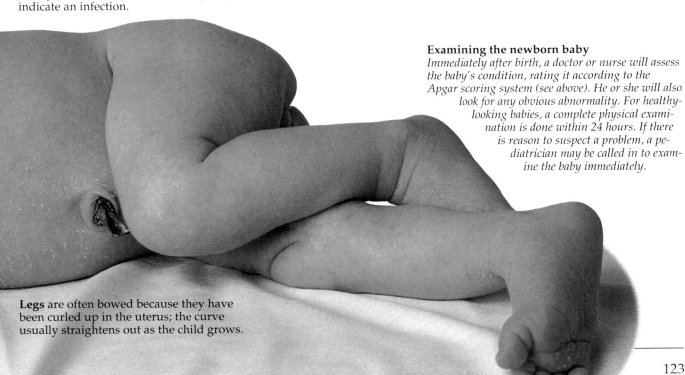

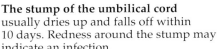

Legs are often bowed because they have been curled up in the uterus; the curve usually straightens out as the child grows.

Skin

At birth, a baby's body (except for the mouth and eyes) is usually covered with a creamy, white substance called vernix, which protected the baby's skin while he or she was in the uterus. The vernix will come off within a few days, but is usually wiped off when the baby is bathed after the birth. The baby's skin may be varied in color – rashes, spots, and blotches are very common during the first month. Tiny, white spots (called "milk spots") may appear on the baby's face, mainly around the nose; these spots will disappear within a few weeks. A blotchy, red rash is very common during the first week and usually disappears within 48 hours. Purple-red patches (known as "stork marks") often occur at the nape of the neck or on the upper eyelids and gradually fade during the first year. Blue-black areas of discoloration over the lower part of the back or the buttocks (known as "mongolian spots") are common in Asian and dark-skinned babies and also fade with time.

Vagina and breasts

Most newborn baby girls have a discharge of mucus, sometimes tinged with blood, from the vagina. The breasts of babies of either sex may become enlarged and secrete a small amount of fluid. These discharges are the result of certain hormones that are passed from the woman to the baby via the placenta and will stop within a week after birth.

BEHAVIOR AND RESPONSES

Newborn babies usually sleep from 15 to 20 hours a day. During those few hours when your new baby is awake, you will notice remarkable responses and patterns of development.

Primitive reflexes
Primitive reflexes are the automatic movements that a newborn baby makes in response to certain stimuli. These reflexes disappear within the first few months as the baby learns to move voluntarily. Examples of primitive reflexes include the grasp reflex (grasping any object that touches the palm of his or her hand) and the walking reflex (a stepping motion triggered by holding the baby upright with the sole of one foot pressed onto a hard surface).

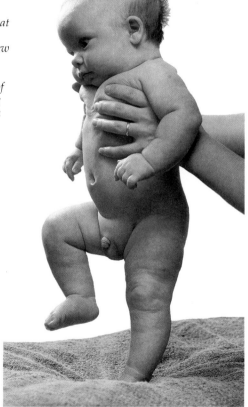

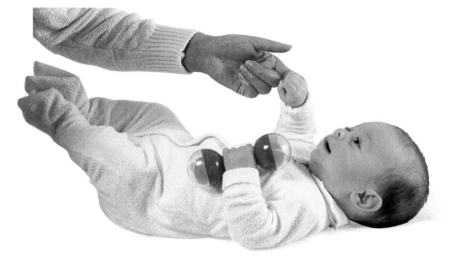

Crying

Most babies cry almost as soon as they are born; birth itself triggers crying to help the baby's lungs function. Crying is the primary way the baby communicates feelings of hunger, thirst, pain, cold, discomfort, and loneliness. Tears rarely appear until the third or fourth week after the baby is born.

Eye movement

Newborn babies are able to distinguish between light and dark but cannot focus on details. Eye movements tend to be wandering and the baby may look cross-eyed at times because of poor muscle coordination during the first few weeks after birth. Newborn babies turn their eyes toward sounds; they seem to prefer the human voice, particularly a high-pitched voice, to other sounds.

Body movement

Newborn babies usually hold their arms and legs in a flexed position. Shaking and twitching movements of a newborn's arms and legs are normal – the baby's nervous system (which controls his or her movements) is still maturing. During the first few months after birth, babies show some involuntary patterns of movements called primitive reflexes (see page 124) in response to certain stimuli.

Feeding and excretion

Most babies can suck and swallow almost as soon as they are born. Just touching an object against the infant's cheek or lips will cause the baby to turn toward the object and start sucking. This response is known as the rooting reflex.

Newborns urinate and pass stools within the first 24 hours. The first stool is a dark brown or green substance called meconium, consisting of swallowed amniotic fluid and mucus from the gastrointestinal tract. The color and consistency of the stools change as the baby starts to eat, becoming a light greenish brown by the third or fourth day.

CIRCUMCISION

Circumcision is the removal of the covering of skin (the foreskin) from the glans (head) of the penis. This procedure is generally safe when performed under sterile conditions by an experienced doctor. Complications are rare but may include bleeding and infection. Talk to your doctor about the possible advantages and potential risks of circumcision, both with and without the use of an anesthetic.

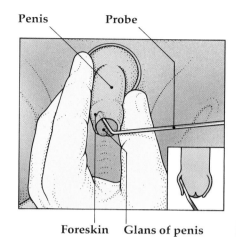

Penis **Probe**

Foreskin **Glans of penis**

1 Using a blunt probe, the foreskin is gently separated from the underlying glans of the penis.

Incision

2 A small incision is made in the foreskin to expose the glans of the penis.

Foreskin

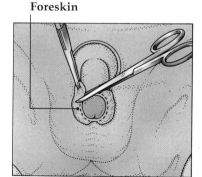

3 The foreskin is pulled back and a portion is cut away with scissors or a scalpel. A specially designed clamp may be used to protect the glans of the penis and help prevent bleeding when the portion of the foreskin is removed.

CIRCUMCISED OR UNCIRCUMCISED?

Research has shown that circumcision decreases the chances of urinary tract infection and reduces the likelihood of inflammation of the head of the penis (a condition called balanitis). A circumcised man may also have a reduced risk of developing cancer of the penis. Female sexual partners of circumcised men seem to have a lower incidence of cancer of the cervix, but the reasons for this are not fully understood.

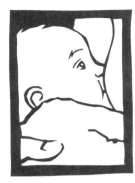

THE POSTPARTUM PERIOD

THE 6 WEEKS AFTER you deliver your baby is called the postpartum period. During this time, your body gradually begins to change back to the way it looked and functioned before your pregnancy. Although you will experience some minor discomforts, eating a sensible diet, getting plenty of rest, and not overdoing it too soon will help ensure a smooth and healthy transition.

While you are in the hospital, your doctor will monitor your condition to make sure you are recovering as you should. He or she will check your temperature, pulse rate, blood pressure, the hemoglobin level in your blood (see page 55), the frequency of bowel movements and how much you urinate, how your uterus is contracting, and the color of your vaginal discharge. Most women go home from the hospital 2 days after delivery (4 days after a cesarean section).

PHYSICAL CHANGES

During your pregnancy, your body will have undergone tremendous changes. Although it will take time for your body to return to normal, the most change occurs during the first 6 weeks after delivery. You will feel better and stronger each day, but it is important that you take time to rest every day and increase your level of activity gradually.

THE FIRST WEEK AFTER DELIVERY

Some of the discomforts that you may experience during the first week after your baby is born are listed below. These are usually a normal part of your body's process of change and recovery. If you are concerned about any signs or symptoms you have after delivery, don't hesitate to call your doctor.

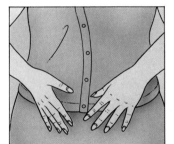

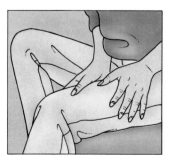

◆ Tiredness
◆ Pains in your abdomen (known as afterpains) as the uterus contracts and moves down from the upper part of the abdomen back into the pelvis
◆ Pain or discomfort in the perineum (the tissue between the vaginal opening and the anus), especially if you had an episiotomy
◆ Discomfort when sitting or walking or a general feeling of soreness in your muscles
◆ A bloody discharge from the vagina

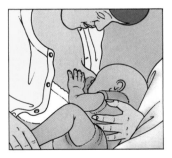

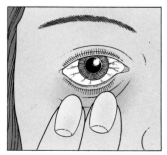

◆ Discomfort when urinating or having a bowel movement
◆ Excessive urination as your body eliminates fluids accumulated during pregnancy
◆ Constipation
◆ Discomfort and enlargement of your breasts; sore nipples if you are breast-feeding your baby
◆ Black-and-blue marks around your eyes or on your cheeks or bloodshot eyes as a result of strenuous pushing during labor and delivery

Changes in the uterus after delivery
Two to 3 days after delivery, the uterus begins to decrease in size. By the end of the first week, it will have shrunk by almost half. The uterus usually returns to about its prepregnancy size in 6 weeks.

Size of uterus before pregnancy

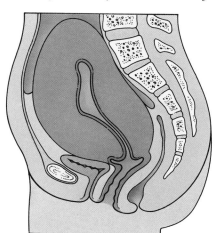

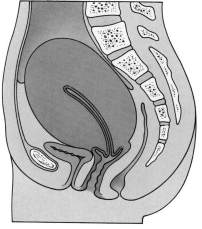

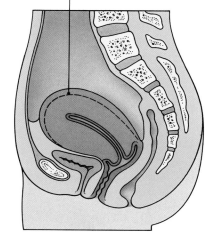

Uterus immediately after childbirth

Uterus 1 week after childbirth

Uterus 6 weeks after childbirth

The cervix
The cervix remains dilated (open) for about 7 to 10 days after delivery. Within 6 weeks, the cervix closes but looks different than it did before pregnancy.

Cervix of a woman who has never had a baby

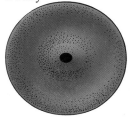

Cervix of a woman who has had a baby

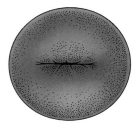

The uterus

The release of hormones after delivery causes the uterus to begin to contract and return toward its normal size (see above). These contractions may cause cramps in the abdomen (known as afterpains). Afterpains may be severe at first but usually subside within 2 or 3 days.

The vagina

Vaginal bleeding (called lochia) is normal after delivery. At first, the discharge is red, usually changing to pink within a week, and then to yellow or brown. The amount of discharge gradually decreases and usually stops within 3 to 6 weeks. If the discharge becomes bright red again or if the amount of discharge suddenly increases, you may be doing too much. Slow down and consult your doctor. If the discharge smells bad or you have a fever, you may have an infection and should call your doctor immediately.

Readjustment of the menstrual cycle after childbirth varies. The first menstrual period usually starts 7 to 9 weeks after childbirth in women who are not breast-feeding. In women who are breast-feeding, levels of the hormones that maintain milk flow delay the first period for as long as breast-feeding continues.

The bladder and bowels

Difficulty urinating during the first few hours after delivery may be caused by the pressure of the uterus on your bladder, an anesthetic you received during labor and delivery, or the discomfort of stitches if you had an episiotomy. It may be necessary to insert a catheter (a thin tube) into your bladder to drain urine. During the first few days after delivery, you will probably urinate more frequently than usual because your body is eliminating excess fluid. Once you go home, if you become unable to urinate, if you experience burning when you urinate, or if your urine becomes cloudy, tinged with blood, or smells bad, call your doctor immediately.

You may not have a bowel movement for 3 to 5 days after delivery. Although physical factors can cause constipation (for example, reduced physical activity and increased elimination of fluids from the body), fear of pain or of splitting episiotomy stitches is also often a factor. To help relieve constipation and ease any discomfort of the first few bowel movements, eat high-fiber foods, drink six to eight glasses of liquids every day, and get up and walk around as often and as soon as possible after delivery.

BREAST-FEEDING

Breast-feeding has potential benefits for both the woman and her baby. It causes an increased release of hormones that help the woman's uterus contract and return toward its normal size more quickly, and breast milk helps the baby's digestion. Breast milk also provides all the nourishment that your baby needs for the first few months and contains substances that help protect him or her against infection and illness. Small, frequent feedings in the first few days help to establish milk flow. Once your milk flow is established, it is important to feed your baby regularly to prevent your breasts from becoming overfilled with milk, which will cause them to become swollen, hard, and painful.

POSITIONS FOR BREAST-FEEDING

You may want to try the breast-feeding positions shown below to determine which works best for you and your baby.

Football hold
Sit in a comfortable chair, placing pillows under your arm on the side you will use to nurse the baby. Hold your baby with this arm, supporting the baby's head and neck with your hand. The baby's body and legs should be tucked under your arm.

Cradle position
Sit in a comfortable chair. Hold your baby in one arm, with his or her head resting in the bend of your arm. You can use a pillow to support your arm and to raise the baby's head up to your breast.

CHOOSING NOT TO BREAST-FEED

Breast-feeding may not be right for all women. You should base this decision on your feelings and desires as well as your life-style. If you choose to bottle-feed your baby, you can be confident that the emotional and physical needs of your baby as well as your own emotional needs will be fulfilled.

Lying down
Lie on your side with a pillow under your head. Lay your baby on his or her side, facing you. A rolled-up blanket placed behind your baby's back will help keep your baby from rolling onto his or her back.

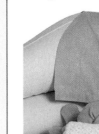

PROBLEMS DURING BREAST-FEEDING

To help relieve sore nipples during the first few weeks, change nursing positions often, nurse frequently so that your baby doesn't get too hungry and suck harder, and make sure all of the nipple is in the baby's mouth. If your breasts become swollen, hard, and sore, you can express (squeeze out) milk and feed it to your baby from a bottle until your nipples are less sore. To help heal cracked skin, avoid using strong soaps and keep your nipples as dry as possible between feedings. A red, tender area may indicate a clogged milk duct. Massaging the breast toward the nipple and continuing to breast-feed usually relieves this problem. Infection can occur if cracking of the skin is severe or if milk backs up in a clogged duct. If you have a warm, sore spot (and possibly a fever), call your doctor immediately.

HOW TO EXPRESS BREAST MILK

1 Place your thumb and fingers behind the areola and squeeze them together while pushing back toward your chest, away from the nipple.

2 Now squeeze toward the nipple. Then move your thumb and fingers a quarter turn and repeat the procedure. Continue until you have gone all the way around your breast.

Milk-producing glands

Milk duct

GETTING YOUR BABY STARTED

If you stroke your baby's cheek, an instinctive reflex causes him or her to turn toward your touch. You can use this reflex to get your baby to start breast-feeding. Touch your nipple to your baby's cheek and move it toward the corner of the baby's mouth. Repeat this several times. The baby will eventually take the nipple into his or her mouth and begin sucking. Be sure your breast does not block the baby's nose and interfere with his or her breathing.

How breast-feeding stimulates milk production
When your baby sucks on the nipple, milk flows from the milk-producing glands at the back of your breasts into tiny sacs called milk ducts under the areola (the dark area surrounding the nipple). The pressure of your baby's mouth on the areola causes milk to be squeezed from the milk ducts out through the nipple. Feeding your baby from one breast at the start of one feeding and then starting from the other breast at the next feeding helps ensure that both breasts receive equal stimulation to produce milk.

129

POSTPARTUM DEPRESSION

About 50 percent of new mothers experience postpartum depression (sometimes called the "baby blues"). Some of the common symptoms are mood swings, irritability, and feelings of loneliness, sadness, and anxiety. Postpartum depression most frequently develops within the first week after delivery and usually lasts for only a few days.

Postpartum depression is believed to be caused by a variety of physical and psychological factors – fatigue, changes in hormone levels, changes in life-style, and personal expectations. After delivery, hormone levels drop dramatically and this fluctuation is believed to trigger depression in some women. Some of the psychological factors that are believed to cause postpartum depression are feelings of anticlimax, uncertainty, and inadequacy; being overwhelmed by new responsibilities; adjustment to no longer being the center of attention; and unhappiness about personal appearance – particularly about weight gained.

Just as there is no specific cause of postpartum depression, there is no "cure" other than the passage of time. Spending time with your partner while the baby is asleep, taking extra care about your appearance, joining an exercise class, or just getting out of the house may help make you feel better.

Most forms of postpartum depression do not require treatment. Some women feel better just talking about their feelings, while others prefer to work through their feelings by themselves. Severe depression is very rare (occurring in less than one in 1,000 women). But, if the depression lasts more than 2 weeks or if you experience sleeplessness, loss of appetite, or feelings of helplessness or hopelessness, you should consult your doctor.

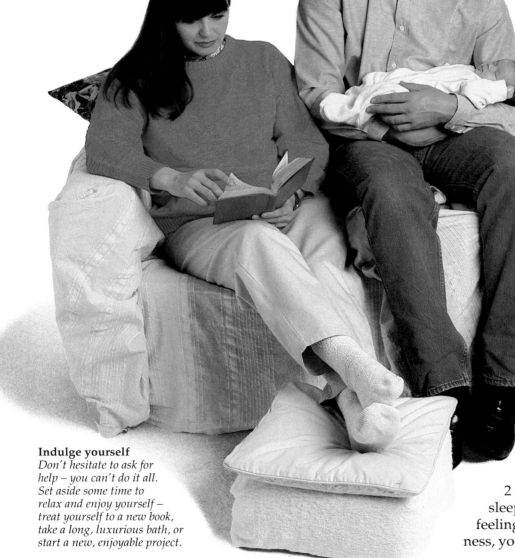

Indulge yourself
Don't hesitate to ask for help – you can't do it all. Set aside some time to relax and enjoy yourself – treat yourself to a new book, take a long, luxurious bath, or start a new, enjoyable project.

STILLBIRTH

A stillbirth is the delivery of a dead fetus after the 28th week of pregnancy. The incidence of stillbirths has decreased dramatically in recent years – from about 19 stillbirths per 1,000 babies born in 1950 to about eight stillbirths per 1,000 babies born in 1985.

CAUSES OF STILLBIRTH

The cause of stillbirth is unknown in about one third of the cases. Some of the possible causes of stillbirth include:

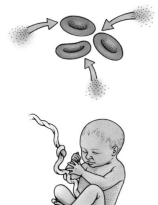

◆ Rh incompatibility (which destroys the fetus's red blood cells – see page 79), severe infections, uncontrolled diabetes, or hypertension (high blood pressure) in the woman or autoimmune disease in the fetus (in which the fetus's immune system attacks the tissues of its own body).

◆ Lack of oxygen to the fetus as a result of the placenta separating from the wall of the uterus; inability of the placenta to provide enough oxygen and nutrients to the fetus; cord prolapse (see page 105); or a knot in the umbilical cord.

◆ Chromosome abnormalities or severe malformations of the fetus.

DIAGNOSIS AND DELIVERY

Death of the fetus is usually diagnosed with electronic monitors that check for the fetus's heartbeat and with ultrasound scanning. When a fetus dies during pregnancy, labor may start spontaneously soon after. If labor does not start on its own, the doctor will induce labor using the drug oxytocin (see page 107).

AFTER THE DELIVERY

Some parents ask for a few private moments alone with the baby. An autopsy is often performed to try to determine the cause of death.

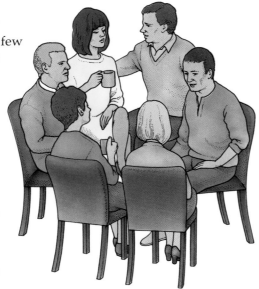

Support and counseling
The sense of loss and grief after a stillbirth can be devastating. The couple often experiences feelings of depression, guilt, anger, and inadequacy. Emotional support from friends and relatives can help the couple cope with their grief. A professional counselor or self-help group may also be useful.

ASK YOUR DOCTOR
POSTPARTUM CARE

Q **Is it true that anything I eat or drink will be passed to my baby through my breast milk?**

A Yes. What you eat or drink while you are breast-feeding can affect the taste of your breast milk. Also, some babies' stomachs are upset by certain foods, such as onions, cabbage, or garlic, so you may want to avoid these items. You should avoid alcohol, too much caffeine, and medications (unless they have been prescribed by your doctor) because these also pass into your breast milk.

Q **Is it true that hemorrhoids often develop during pregnancy? If so, why does it happen and how is this problem treated?**

A Hemorrhoids (swollen veins in and around the anus) can develop during pregnancy. They are often caused by the pressure of the enlarged uterus. Hemorrhoids usually shrink within a month after delivery. Warm baths and drinking six to eight glasses of liquids a day and eating high-fiber foods to avoid constipation may help relieve the discomfort. Talk to your doctor before using any cream or suppositories.

Q **I had my baby 4 weeks ago. How long should I wait before having sexual intercourse?**

A Most doctors advise couples to abstain from sexual intercourse until after the first checkup following childbirth (usually at 6 weeks). If you haven't had your first menstrual period before you have intercourse, you should use some form of birth control because conception can occur regardless of whether your menstrual cycle has started again.

CHAPTER FIVE

INFERTILITY

INTRODUCTION

CAUSES OF
INFERTILITY

TESTING AND
TREATMENT

IN RECENT YEARS, the number of infertile couples in the US has risen by about 30 percent. Various social factors are believed to have contributed to this increase – more women are now in their childbearing years, couples are marrying later in life, and women are delaying childbearing until their mid-30s. Also, there is greater overall awareness of infertility problems. An infertility problem affects one in every seven couples – about 15 percent of adults. The numbers of infertile men and women are about equal. Infertility can be caused by external factors (such as stress, life-style, or environmental hazards) or by internal problems (such as abnormalities in hormone levels or in the function or structure of the reproductive system). Extensive evaluation, examination, testing, and treatment may be needed. The cause of infertility can be determined in about 90 percent of cases.

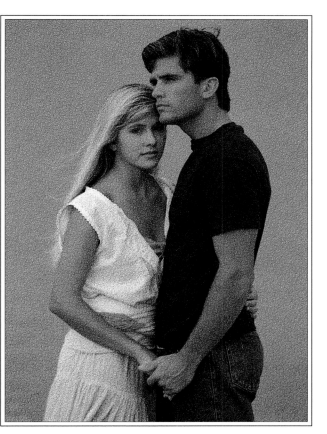

Continuing progress in our understanding of the reproductive process and the causes of infertility, advances in medical technology, and the development of ever more sophisticated drug treatments have led to the availability of an array of treatments for infertility problems. Better understanding of the actions of hormones has enabled doctors to both control and stimulate ovulation. The first successful fertility drug was clomiphene, which stimulates the release of eggs from the ovaries. This major breakthrough was followed by the use of follicle-stimulating hormone (FSH), which has a more powerful stimulant effect than clomiphene. Laparoscopic surgery and ultrasound scanning have also helped to improve the diagnosis and treatment of infertility. These techniques paved the way for in vitro fertilization (the fertilization of an egg in the laboratory). In vitro fertilization and related techniques for implantation of a fertilized egg that have recently been developed have helped thousands of women to conceive who had previously been unable to have a baby. Fertility specialists can offer advice, counseling, support, and treatment to many couples. Couples who choose to undergo fertility treatments must consider how much of themselves they can afford to invest emotionally, physically, and financially. Although fertility treatments provide a childless couple with new hope, both partners must remember that, for any month of treatment, failure is more likely than success. Although 35 to 40 percent of infertile couples today never conceive, continuing advances in fertility treatments promise ever greater chances of achieving pregnancy.

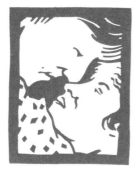

CAUSES OF INFERTILITY

A COUPLE WHO HAS BEEN HAVING unprotected sexual intercourse around the time of ovulation each menstrual cycle for at least 1 year and has been unable to conceive may have a fertility problem. In women, abnormalities of the reproductive tract are common causes of infertility. In men, the most common cause of infertility is failure to produce enough healthy sperm.

PELVIC INFLAMMATORY DISEASE

Pelvic inflammatory disease, an infection of a woman's internal reproductive organs, may cause infertility as a result of blockage or scarring of tissues, which can prevent sperm from reaching the egg. The infection often occurs after a sexually transmitted disease, such as chlamydial infection or gonorrhea. Women who use an intrauterine device (an IUD) or who have numerous sexual partners have an increased risk of developing pelvic inflammatory disease.

About 40 percent of cases of infertility are caused by problems in the woman and 30 percent are caused by problems in the man. In about 30 percent of cases, both partners have a fertility problem.

THE RANGE OF PROBLEMS

There are many possible causes of infertility. The problem in the woman may be the inability of the ovaries to produce mature eggs or a blockage in or damage to the fallopian tubes. In the man, the sperm may be defective or there may be a problem in the reproductive tract (such as blockage of tubes connecting the testicles, where sperm are produced, and the urethra, through which sperm are ejaculated). Infertility problems may also be caused by various abnormalities of hormone production, sexual dysfunctions (such as impotence – the inability to achieve or maintain an erection), or social and life-style factors (such as excessive smoking or consumption of alcohol).

FEMALE FERTILITY PROBLEMS

Problems with egg release

 Anovulation (in which mature eggs are not released by the ovaries) and irregular release of eggs from the ovaries are the most common causes of infertility in women. These problems are the result of hormone imbalances, which may be caused by excessive weight loss, obesity, or, in some cases, polycystic ovarian disease (in which cysts develop in the ovaries).

Blocked or damaged fallopian tubes

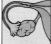 The fallopian tubes may be damaged or blocked as a result of infection, surgery on the pelvic organs, or a condition called endometriosis (see below). This blockage or damage may prevent sperm from reaching the egg or may prevent a fertilized egg from moving through the fallopian tube into the uterus.

Abnormalities of the uterus

 In rare cases, abnormalities of the uterus cause infertility. The uterus may not have formed properly, scar tissue (resulting from surgery or infection) may block all or part of the uterine cavity, or fibroids (noncancerous tumors) may distort the shape of the uterus.

Problems of the cervix

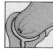 A hormone imbalance can make the mucus of the cervix impermeable to sperm. The sperm are unable to travel through the cervix toward the fallopian tubes to fertilize an egg.

Endometriosis

Endometriosis is a condition in which fragments of tissue that may have been shed from the lining of the uterus (the endometrium) adhere to and grow on organs in the abdomen. This tissue responds to hormones in the same way as does the endometrium – it bleeds during menstruation. The bleeding can cause scar tissue to form that may block the fallopian tubes, leading to infertility.

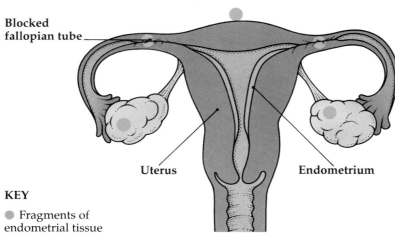

Blocked fallopian tube

Uterus   Endometrium

KEY
● Fragments of endometrial tissue

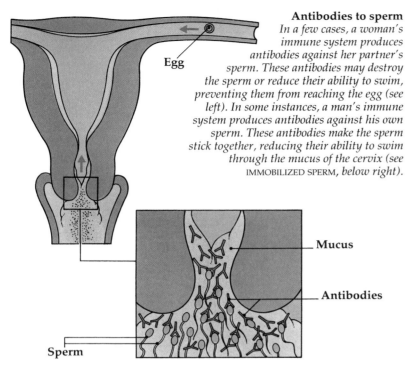

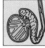

Egg

Mucus

Antibodies

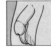

Sperm

Antibodies to sperm
In a few cases, a woman's immune system produces antibodies against her partner's sperm. These antibodies may destroy the sperm or reduce their ability to swim, preventing them from reaching the egg (see left). In some instances, a man's immune system produces antibodies against his own sperm. These antibodies make the sperm stick together, reducing their ability to swim through the mucus of the cervix (see IMMOBILIZED SPERM, *below right).*

MALE INFERTILITY PROBLEMS

Abnormal sperm production
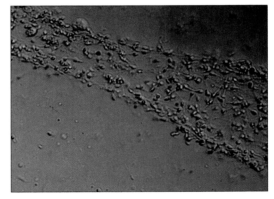

The most common cause of infertility in men is a low sperm count (a lower-than-normal production of sperm). Infertility can also occur if too many of the sperm that are produced are defective. Of the millions of sperm that are normally produced in the testicles every day, about 20 percent are defective in some way. If the proportion of abnormal sperm is unusually high, the likelihood of fertilization occurring will be reduced. Such problems with sperm production may be caused by hormone abnormalities, illness, medications, use of illegal drugs, or excessive consumption of alcohol.

Problems with the passage of sperm

The sperm must pass through tubular structures – the epididymis and then the vas deferens – to reach the penis. If these structures become blocked as a result of infection or if they have not developed properly, sperm may be unable to pass through, resulting in infertility.

Problems of ejaculation

Structural abnormalities of the ejaculatory duct (see page 14) may reduce or prevent ejaculation of sperm from the penis. Damage to nerves, sometimes resulting from surgery on the prostate gland, may lead to sperm being ejaculated backward into the bladder. Some types of medications or severe damage to the spine can affect the nerve signals that trigger ejaculation.

Hope for infertile couples?
Infertility does not necessarily mean that a couple's dreams of becoming parents must be forgotten. With treatments such as fertility drugs, artificial insemination (see page 140), and in vitro fertilization (see page 141), many previously infertile couples are able to have a baby.

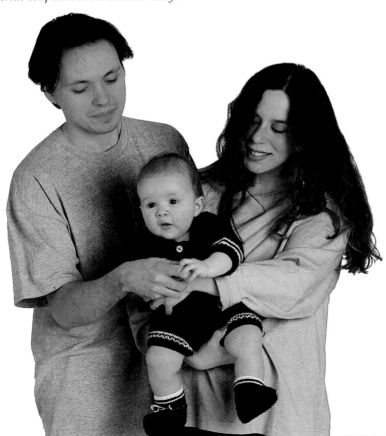

Immobilized sperm
Following a vasectomy, a sterilization operation in which each vas deferens (the two tubes through which sperm pass from the testicles) is cut and then stitched closed or tied off, the man's immune system may produce antibodies that cause the sperm to stick together (as shown above, magnified 100 times). If the operation is subsequently reversed, the reduced mobility of the sperm as a result of these antibodies may cause infertility.

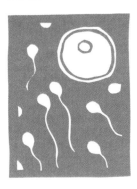

TESTING AND TREATMENT

MOST DOCTORS ADVISE couples to try to conceive for at least 1 year before seeking professional help for infertility. Both partners may undergo tests to try to determine the cause of the problem. If possible, the doctor will treat the cause of the infertility. If treatment is not successful, he or she may recommend procedures such as in vitro fertilization to achieve pregnancy.

When seeking professional help for an infertility problem, talk to your family doctor or gynecologist first because the problem can sometimes be solved simply – for example, by changing the timing of sexual intercourse. If no obvious cause can be found or if the cause requires specialized treatment, your doctor may recommend an infertility specialist. An infertility evaluation usually begins with thorough physical examinations of both partners. The doctor will ask questions about your medical history, how long you have been trying to become pregnant, previous use of contraception and whether you have been pregnant before, and the frequency and timing of intercourse. The doctor may then recommend a series of tests.

TESTING FOR FEMALE INFERTILITY

The doctor pursues three main areas in testing the female partner – whether eggs are being released from the ovaries (the process called ovulation) and whether this release occurs regularly every month, whether there are abnormalities of the uterus or fallopian tubes (see page 137), and whether there is a problem with the mucus of the cervix that may be preventing the penetration of sperm. Failure to ovulate is the most common cause of female infertility.

Various changes in a woman's body can help indicate if and when ovulation is occurring. For example, after ovulation, the body temperature increases slightly; a daily record of a woman's body temperature can be used to detect this increase (see page 22). Changes in the lining of the uterus (the endometrium) also occur after ovulation. The endometrium becomes thickened as the blood supply to vessels in the lining increases and glands in the lining enlarge. The doctor can detect these changes by examining a sample of tissue from the endometrium under a microscope. Ultrasound scanning (see page 58) can be used to detect changes in the size of a follicle (which contains the egg). As the follicle matures in the ovary, it increases in size and then gets smaller after ovulation.

"Stretchable" cervical mucus

Fern pattern formed when mucus dries

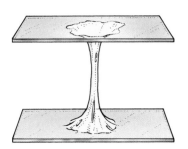

Examining cervical mucus
Just before ovulation, the mucus of the cervix becomes more "stretchable." To check for this change in the mucus, a sample is placed between two glass slides; the slides are then slowly separated to check how the mucus stretches (see above left). The cervical mucus that is normally secreted just before ovulation shows a characteristic fern pattern when dried on a glass slide (see above right).

Measurements of hormone levels in the blood or urine over a period of time can also help detect ovulation. Before ovulation, levels of luteinizing hormone (LH) and follicle-stimulating hormone (FSH) increase in the blood and urine; after ovulation, the level of progesterone in the blood increases. Your doctor may recommend that you use an ovulation kit (available in most drugstores) to help determine when ovulation is about to occur. These kits detect high levels of LH in a urine sample.

Changes in the mucus of the cervix may prevent sperm from entering the uterus. Around the time of ovulation, the doctor may take a sample of the cervical mucus a few hours after a woman has had intercourse. The sample is examined under a microscope to check the number of sperm and their movement.

TESTING FOR MALE INFERTILITY

When trying to determine the cause of infertility in the male partner, the doctor analyzes a sample of semen. The quantity of semen and the number of sperm in a specified amount of semen are measured, and the movement and shape of the sperm are assessed. The doctor also checks for signs of infection.

If sperm are not being produced or the number of sperm is unusually low, measurements of hormone levels in the blood can help to identify the cause of the problem. For example, high blood levels of follicle-stimulating hormone (FSH) indicate an abnormality in the testicles. Normal levels of FSH suggest that the testicles are producing sperm but the tubes through which sperm pass from the testicles are blocked. A biopsy (the removal of tissue for examination under a microscope) of the testicles may be done to confirm this diagnosis.

Failure to produce sperm or an unusually low sperm count is sometimes the result of a chromosome abnormality. This

EXAMINING THE UTERUS AND FALLOPIAN TUBES

Two techniques, hysterosalpingography and laparoscopy (see below), are often used to check for abnormalities of the uterus and/or the fallopian tubes.

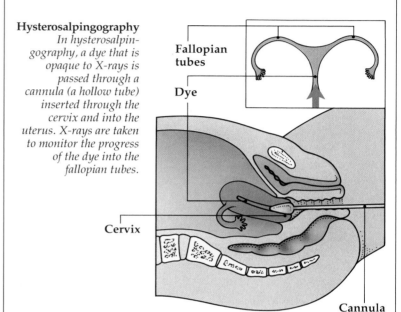

Hysterosalpingography
In hysterosalpingography, a dye that is opaque to X-rays is passed through a cannula (a hollow tube) inserted through the cervix and into the uterus. X-rays are taken to monitor the progress of the dye into the fallopian tubes.

Fallopian tubes

Dye

Cervix

Cannula

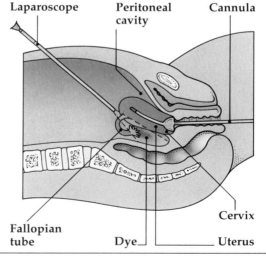

Laparoscope

Peritoneal cavity

Cannula

Fallopian tube

Dye

Cervix

Uterus

Laparoscopy
Through a small incision in the abdomen, the doctor inserts a viewing tube called a laparoscope into the peritoneal cavity (which contains the uterus). Dye is passed through a cannula inserted through the cervix and into the uterus. The doctor watches through the laparoscope to check that the dye flows out through the ends of the fallopian tubes.

type of abnormality can be detected by analyzing the chromosomes in white blood cells taken from a blood sample. A blood sample can also be analyzed for antibodies to sperm, which may be a cause of defective sperm.

TREATING FEMALE INFERTILITY

Treatment of anovulation (the absence of egg release by the ovaries) depends on the cause of the problem. If the cause of anovulation is excessive exercise or being severely underweight, reducing the amount of exercise or increasing body weight to a normal level may allow ovulation to resume. If these measures are not successful, the doctor may recommend treatment with fertility drugs to stimulate ovulation (see right). Anovulation that is the result of a severe illness may also be treated with fertility drugs. If high levels of the hormone prolactin in the blood are the cause of anovulation, drugs such as bromocriptine may be given to inhibit prolactin production, which may restore ovulation.

Surgical treatment

In many cases, blockage of or damage to fallopian tubes can be treated surgically. When only one section of the fallopian tube has become narrowed or blocked, techniques called tubal reanastomosis

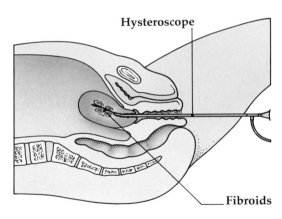

Treating uterine fibroids
In a few cases, uterine fibroids (noncancerous tumors) cause infertility – for example, if they are very large or are located so that they prevent implantation of a fertilized egg. Fibroids can sometimes be treated with medication, but surgery may be necessary. If fibroids protrude into the cavity of the uterus, surgical removal can be done using an instrument called a hysteroscope (see above). Abdominal surgery is required to remove fibroids on the outside of the uterus.

FERTILITY DRUGS

Fertility drugs are effective in most women. These drugs can be used in two ways to stimulate ovulation (see below). Treatment with fertility drugs is carefully monitored because these drugs can cause release of several eggs at one time, leading to a multiple pregnancy (more than one fetus). A multiple pregnancy poses an increased risk for both the woman and the fetuses.

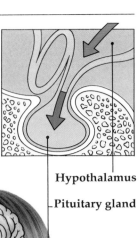

Hypothalamus
Pituitary gland

KEY
- Clomiphene
- GnRH
- FSH
- LH

Indirect stimulation of the ovary
The drug clomiphene stimulates an area in the brain called the hypothalamus to increase production of gonadotropin-releasing hormone (GnRH), which in turn stimulates the release of follicle-stimulating hormone (FSH) and luteinizing hormone (LH) from the pituitary gland. FSH and LH stimulate the ovaries.

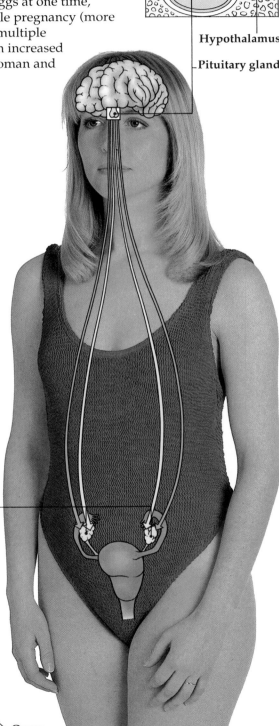

Ovaries

Direct stimulation of the ovaries
The ovaries can also be directly stimulated by giving GnRH or FSH and LH.

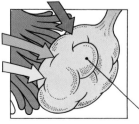

Ovary

and tuboplasty may be used to restore fertility (see below). Blockage of the end of a fallopian tube closest to the ovary can be treated using a technique called salpingostomy (see below). Salpingolysis is a technique used if fertilization is being prevented by adhesions (abnormal tissue connections) that have formed between fallopian tubes and surrounding tissues (see below). These adhesions may be caused by infection of organs within the abdomen or previous abdominal or pelvic surgery. If a blocked or damaged fallopian tube cannot be repaired surgically, the doctor may recommend trying in vitro fertilization (see page 141).

The risk of ectopic pregnancy (implantation of a fertilized egg outside the uterus, including in a fallopian tube) may be increased as a result of surgery on the fallopian tube. If an ectopic pregnancy develops, surgery to terminate the pregnancy may further reduce the chances of conception.

Tubal reanastomosis
This procedure is used when only one section of the fallopian tube is blocked. The doctor removes the narrowed section of the fallopian tube and then stitches the ends of the remaining two parts of the tube together.

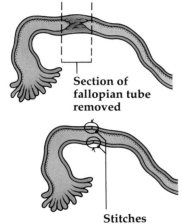

Section of fallopian tube removed

Stitches

Salpingolysis
A technique called salpingolysis can be used to remove adhesions. Adhesions are abnormal tissue connections between a fallopian tube and other tissues that can distort the fallopian tube. The adhesions are either cut away with a scalpel or broken down with a laser beam.

Adhesions

Laser beam

Distorted fallopian tube

Salpingostomy
This procedure (right) may be used when the outer end of the fallopian tube has become blocked. The fimbriae (finger-like projections) at the end of the tube are opened outward. The edges of the tube's opening are turned slightly down and stitched to prevent reclosure of the tube.

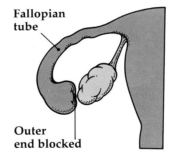

Fallopian tube

Outer end blocked

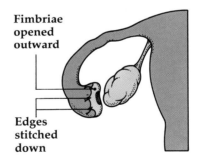

Fimbriae opened outward

Edges stitched down

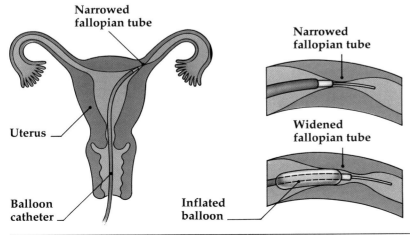

Narrowed fallopian tube

Uterus

Balloon catheter

Narrowed fallopian tube

Widened fallopian tube

Inflated balloon

Tuboplasty
This technique may be done to treat a blocked or narrowed fallopian tube. A small balloon-tipped tube called a balloon catheter is inserted through the uterus and into the fallopian tube (top left). The balloon is inflated to widen or unblock the tube (bottom left). The balloon is then deflated and the catheter is withdrawn.

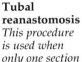

TREATING ANTIBODIES TO SPERM
When infertility is the result of a woman's immune system producing antibodies against her partner's sperm, the doctor may recommend using a condom for 2 to 3 months so the woman's immune system will not be exposed to the sperm and produce antibodies against them. After this time, if unprotected sexual intercourse around the time of ovulation does not result in pregnancy, artificial insemination (see page 140) or in vitro fertilization (see page 141) may be recommended. If a man's immune system is producing antibodies against his own sperm, the doctor may prescribe drugs that suppress responses of the immune system to help reduce antibody production. In some cases, antibodies against sperm can be washed from a sample of semen; the washed semen is then inserted into the woman's uterus by artificial insemination.

TREATING MALE INFERTILITY

In some cases of male infertility, the most effective treatment involves self-help measures to improve general health, such as eating a nutritious diet, stopping smoking, cutting down alcohol consumption, and reducing stress.

Treatment with fertility drugs is sometimes effective for improving a low sperm count. If the infertility problem is the result of a failure of the testicles to produce sperm, injections of gonadotropins (hormones that stimulate cell activity in the testicles) may be given.

Abnormalities in the sperm or semen may be the result of an infection of the prostate gland or other structures that produce semen. Such problems are sometimes resolved after treatment with antibiotic drugs to clear up the infection.

Surgical treatment

Surgery can sometimes correct structural abnormalities that are causing infertility; for example, a blockage in the vas deferens (the tube that connects each testicle to the urethra) can be removed. If a man who has had a vasectomy (an operation in which each vas deferens is cut) wants his fertility restored, a procedure to reverse the vasectomy is successful about 50 percent of the time.

TREATING UNEXPLAINED INFERTILITY

Some couples are unable to conceive despite normal results of fertility tests and having unprotected sexual intercourse every other day for the 4- to 5-day period surrounding the time of ovulation. Fertility drugs, artificial insemination, and in vitro fertilization may be tried.

ARTIFICIAL INSEMINATION

When a woman is artificially inseminated, sperm (from the woman's partner or from a donor) are inserted into the cervix. The procedure is performed around the time of ovulation. Fertility drugs are sometimes given to help improve the chances of fertilization. Artificial insemination may be done if the cause of infertility cannot be determined, if

antibodies to sperm (see page 135) are produced, if abnormalities of the cervix (see page 134) have prevented sperm from entering the uterus, or if sexual intercourse is not possible. The success rate of artificial insemination varies between about 20 percent after the first attempt to about 80 percent at the end of the sixth attempt.

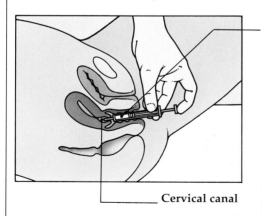

Syringe containing semen

Cervical canal

How artificial insemination is done
The semen is inserted into the cervical canal using a small syringe. The woman remains lying on her back for 20 minutes after the procedure.

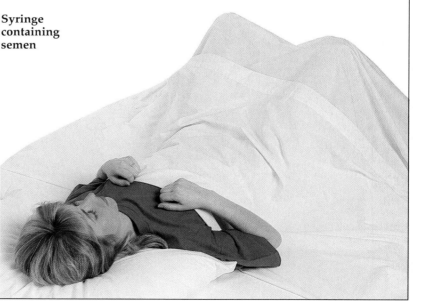

IN VITRO FERTILIZATION

In vitro fertilization (IVF) involves the joining of eggs with sperm outside the woman's body. IVF may be done if the cause of infertility cannot be determined, if antibodies to sperm (see page 139) are produced, if a woman has blocked or damaged fallopian tubes that cannot be treated, or if a couple is unable to have sexual intercourse. The rate of successful pregnancies (commonly referred to as "take-home babies") from each IVF attempt ranges between 15 and 20 percent.

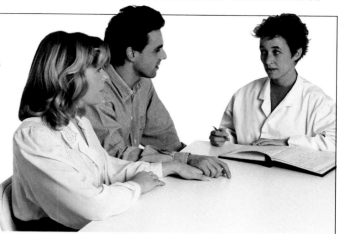

1 Before treatment is started, the doctor explains the techniques that will be involved, the chances of success, and any possible risks.

2 Fertility drugs are usually given to stimulate several eggs to mature in the ovaries. The growth of the follicles (which contain the eggs) is monitored by ultrasound scanning and measurement of certain hormone levels in the blood that increase as the eggs mature (see page 12). When the eggs are almost mature, the woman is given an injection of the hormone human chorionic gonadotropin (HCG), which stimulates the ovaries to produce estrogen and progesterone – hormones needed to maintain a pregnancy.

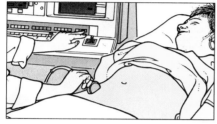

Ultrasound transducer

3 Immediately before ovulation, the doctor removes the eggs, using either laparoscopy (see page 87) or ultrasound-guided needle aspiration (see right). With the latter technique, the ultrasound probe allows the doctor to see the positioning of the needle on a monitor.

Ovary containing mature eggs

Ultrasound probe　　**Aspiration needle**

4 To fertilize the eggs, they are mixed with the sperm, placed under domes in a culture dish, and put in an incubator.

Domes covering eggs and sperm

NEW DEVELOPMENTS

Two new procedures – known as GIFT and ZIFT – may help couples with an unexplained infertility problem. These procedures were developed based on the theory that conception is most likely to occur when the egg and sperm are placed in the environment where fertilization naturally occurs – the fallopian tube. In GIFT (gamete intrafallopian transfer), mature eggs (called gametes) are collected using the same technique as for in vitro fertilization. The eggs are then mixed with sperm and placed into the fallopian tube. ZIFT (zygote intrafallopian transfer) involves placing an egg that has already been fertilized (called a zygote) in a laboratory into the fallopian tube. The rate of successful pregnancies for both GIFT and ZIFT ranges between 20 and 25 percent.

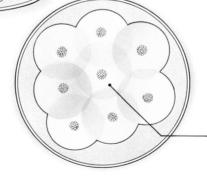

5 Each fertilized egg is transferred to a separate culture dish. When the eggs have grown to about eight cells, they have become embryos and are ready to be transferred to the uterus.

Embryo ready for transfer

6 The embryos are drawn up into a catheter (a thin tube). The catheter is inserted through the cervix, and four or five embryos are placed in the uterus. The doctor may give the woman an additional injection of HCG.

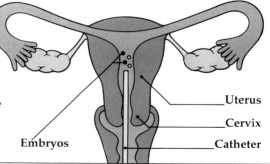

Uterus

Cervix

Catheter

Embryos

Photograph sources:
Bubbles Photo Library **66** (top); **100**
Robert Harding Photo Library **44**
Sally Hill, Ultrasound Diagnostic Services **68** (bottom left)
The Image Bank **9**; **27** (top left); **47**; **78**; **133**
Lupe Cunha Photo Library **124**
National Blood Transfusion Services **57**
Northwestern Memorial Hospital **50**
NURTURE **135** (bottom right)
The Photographers' Library **25**
Pictor International Ltd **65** (center)
Reflections Photo Library **67**
Science Photo Library **2** (bottom right); **15**; **16** (top right); **16** (bottom right); **20** (bottom); **30**; **32**; **59**; **72**; **83**; **120** (top)

Tony Stone Worldwide **7**; **89**
Dr A.Walker **136**
Dr J. Zakrzewska, Eastman Dental Hospital **64**
Zefa **82**

Front cover photograph:
Stephen Marks/Stockphotos

Maternity wear supplied by:
Bumpsadaisy, 52 Chiltern Street, London W1, UK

Illustrators:
Tony Bellue
Karen Cochrane
David Fathers
Tony Graham
Andrew Green
Coral Mula
Lydia Umney
Philip Wilson
John Woodcock

Commissioned photography:
Susannah Price

Airbrushing:
Janos Marffy

Index:
Sue Bosanko